THE TEACHING
FUNCTION
OF THE NURSING
PRACTITIONER

FOUNDATIONS OF NURSING SERIES

WM. C. BROWN COMPANY PUBLISHERS

Nursing Observation
Virginia B. Byers
University of Pittsburgh

Nursing Observations of the Young Patient
Margaret A. Coffin
Boston University, School of Nursing

Promotion of Physical Comfort and Safety, Second Edition
Valentina G. Fischer, Columbia University
Arlene F. Connolly, Boston University, School of Nursing

Promoting Psychological Comfort, Second Edition
Gloria M. Francis and Barbara Munjas
Virginia Commonwealth University

Problem Solving in Nursing Practice, Second Edition
Mae M. Johnson, Los Angeles Valley College
Mary Lou C. Davis

Nurse-Patient Communication
Garland K. Lewis
The Catholic University of America

Working with Others for Patient Care
Grace G. Peterson
DePaul University

The Teaching Function of the Nursing Practitioner
Margaret L. Pohl
Hunter College

Planning Patient Care
Lucile Lewis
Loma Linda University

Second Edition

THE TEACHING FUNCTION OF THE NURSING PRACTITIONER

Margaret L. Pohl

Formerly Assistant Professor of Nursing Education
Hunter College of the City University of New York

WM. C. BROWN COMPANY PUBLISHERS, *Dubuque, Iowa*

Contents

Preface   vii

1. Teaching as a Function of Nursing   1

Definition of Terms   1
The Importance of the Practitioner's Teaching Function   3
Opportunities for Teaching in Nursing   3
A Basic Premise about the Practitioner's Teaching   4
A Note about Reference Readings in *this* Book   4

2. Principles of Learning   6

Definition of Principles   6
Application of Principles   7
Principles of Learning and Their Applications
    to Nursing   7
Summary   24

3. Principles of Teaching   26

The Source of Teaching Principles   26
Principles of Teaching in Nursing Settings   27
Summary   39

4. The Learners   42

Factors in Nursing Settings that Affect Teaching
    and Learning   42
Patients in Various Stages of Illness   43
Patients Who Have Problems in Communicating   48

Clients in Good Health   54
Co-Workers Supervised by the Practitioner   57
Co-Workers in Schools and Industry   58
Summary   59

5. **The Subject Matter**   62

Content Related to Health Status   62
Content Related to Giving Nursing Care   65
Content Related to the Orientation of New Workers   67
Summary   68

6. **Methods of Teaching**   70

Informal Teaching   70
Structured Teaching   73
Teaching Through Supervision   80
Summary   84

7. **Teaching Materials**   87

General Considerations   87
Types of Teaching Materials   89
Devices for Displaying Teaching Materials   94
Sources of Teaching Materials   97
Summary   100

8. **Planning for Teaching**   102

Planning the Overall Teaching Program   102
Preparing Teaching Guides   105
An Example of a Teaching Guide   109
Summary   110

9. **Evaluating Teaching and Learning**   115

General Considerations   115
Objectivity and Subjectivity   116
Evaluation and Objectives   118
Evaluating the Learning of Clients and Co-Workers   118
Evaluating the Co-Worker's Nursing Care   119
Self-Evaluation   121
Evaluating the Total Teaching Program   123
Summary   124

Index   127

Preface

This book was written to assist graduate nursing practitioners to teach a variety of people what they may need to know about health and illness, and to introduce students of nursing to this area of the nurse's responsibility.

In this second edition, the original content has been reorganized, new subject matter has been added, and the reference readings have been revised. As heretofore, emphasis in the readings remains on annotated articles from nursing journals on the assumption that such sources would be available to most readers. Certain readings suggested in the first edition have been repeated because of their relevance to specific aspects of the subject matter. However, with the exception of Gilbert Highet's 1954 classic, *The Art of Teaching*, all references were published in 1960 or thereafter.

The importance of communication as an essential factor in teaching and learning has been stressed, and a new section added concerning patients who have problems in communicating. More emphasis has been placed on the convalescent period as a time of inner stress that the nurse may overlook, and as a period for effective teaching and learning if this stress can be allayed.

A new chapter has been added on evaluating teaching and learning. The material on this topic has been assembled from various chapters in the earlier edition and expanded to include discussions of objectivity, subjectivity, and self-evaluation for both teacher and learner.

The author would like to express appreciation for the editorial assistance given again by Dr. Eleanor M. Schetlin and for the typing of the manuscript by Mrs. Nita Sell.

PREFACE TO THE FIRST EDITION

This book was written to assist present and future nursing practitioners to teach patients, families, and auxiliary nursing personnel what they may need to know about health and illness. It is intended for use in programs that prepare nursing practitioners, in inservice programs for graduate nurses, and for individual study by nurses who want to improve their teaching ability. The need for more adequate preparation of nurses in this area was revealed in a study conducted by the author (Margaret L. Pohl, "A Study of the Teaching Activities of the Nursing Practitioner," Doctor of Education Project Report, New York, Teachers College, Columbia University, 1963) in which the teaching activities of 1,500 nursing practitioners throughout the United States were surveyed. Almost all of these nurses reported a need for teaching skills, but over 900 stated that their preparation for teaching was either lacking or inadequate for their purposes as practicing graduate nurses. It is hoped that this book will meet the need for a text on teaching specifically designed for practitioners in various nursing settings, and for those preparing to become practitioners.

A fundamental premise of this book is that nursing practitioners have a social and professional responsibility to promote good health practices by meeting the health learning needs of patients, families, and nursing assistants; at the same time, it is recognized that teaching is only one aspect of the nurse's total obligation and that other functions may often take priority over teaching.

Basic principles of learning and teaching are presented and applications are made to the nursing settings in which the practitioner may function: hospitals, clinics, homes, schools, health services in business and industry, and physicians' offices. Problems of learning and teaching peculiar to these situations are considered; content, methods, and materials that might be used are focused specifically on what would be appropriate in such settings. The final chapter includes suggestions for the preliminary planning and continual evaluation of the practitioner's teaching, and presents a teaching guide that could be adapted for use in a variety of circumstances.

Annotated readings are suggested to add further illustrations of the application of general principles; many of the references have been selected from nursing journals published since 1960, on the assumption that they would be available to most readers.

The author would like to express appreciation for the assistance given by Dr. Eleanor M. Schetlin in editing the material in this book and by Mrs. Jean Meeker in typing the manuscript for publication.

Chapter ———— 1

Teaching as a Function of Nursing

This book is concerned with the teaching function of the nursing practitioner. The basic purpose of nursing is the promotion of health; teaching is one of the nurse's activities that contributes to the attainment of that aim. Regardless of whether the practitioner works in the hospital, the home, the doctor's office, or a health service in school or industry, the goal of nursing is to provide the comprehensive care that will improve and maintain the best health possible for the members of our society. To accomplish this purpose, nurses must be able to apply their knowledge and skill in carrying out the many responsibilities that make up their total nursing function. These activities include giving physical care to the patient; helping him, directly or indirectly, to meet his emotional, social, and spiritual needs; assisting his family and others with their health problems; cooperating with physicians and other professional people in their plans for the patient; directing the work of nonprofessional nursing personnel; assuming responsibility for health supervision; and teaching a variety of individuals and groups about health and illness. The effective performance of these functions constitutes the practice of nursing; effective teaching is an essential part of this practice.

DEFINITION OF TERMS

In order to clarify the scope and the limitations of the content of this book, definition of certain terms is necessary at the outset.

The Nursing Practitioner, the Nurse

Throughout this book, these terms will be used to refer to the student of nursing or the registered nurse who is employed in giving direct nursing service. This service includes both the bedside care and the health supervision of many kinds of people who have direct contact with the nurse in many different settings. Thus, we are not concerned here with the activities of nurses who are faculty members, supervisors, or administrators of nursing services, but only with the men and women who are or will be registered nurses working directly with the people for whom nursing service is being provided.

The Teaching Function

This term will be used to mean the sum of all the activities by which the practitioner helps the learner to understand and apply knowledge about health and illness. The term includes informal activities as well as more structured teaching.

There is an important difference between the teacher in a school setting and the nursing practitioner as a teacher. The primary concern of the school teacher is education and all the teacher's time is devoted to this goal; the primary concern of the nurse is nursing service, and teaching is only one aspect of many responsibilities. Therefore, the practitioner's teaching must bear a reasonable relationship to other nursing functions. The nurse must evaluate every situation to determine priorities. When the patient is acutely ill, it is obvious that teaching must be delayed until his physical needs have been met. With patients who are convalescing and with people in good health, teaching often assumes priority. Thus, the practitioner is not a teacher as such, but has a teaching function.

Clients

This term will refer to all the people to whom the practitioner gives direct nursing service, regardless of the state of their health. The term, therefore, includes both patients and people who are well. It is customary to speak of clients in relation to the practice of law or social work, rather than in relation to nursing. However, the term will be used in this book to avoid the awkward phrase "patients and people who are well" when reference is made collectively to all the people to whom the nurse gives direct nursing care or health supervision.

Co-workers

The use of this term will be limited to the co-workers for whom the practitioner has a teaching responsibility. This limitation is necessary because many of the nurse's co-workers are professionally educated people who are thoroughly grounded in the principles and practices of good health and therefore have no need for the practitioner's teaching.

There are two groups of co-workers whom the nurse *does* teach. One group includes the nursing personnel whose work the practitioner supervises; for example, practical nurses and nursing assistants in hospitals and other health agencies. The second group includes people in schools and industry who have some responsibility for the health of pupils or employees; for example, teachers in schools and supervisors in industry.

The term will not be used to mean physicians, professional workers in allied fields, or nurses who administer or supervise nursing services, since, although they are co-workers, the practitioner does not have responsibility for teaching them.

THE IMPORTANCE OF THE PRACTITIONER'S TEACHING FUNCTION

If the goal of optimum health is to be realized, the cooperation of the members of our society is essential. People must be helped through education to assume responsibility for their own health and the health of family members who are unable to do so for themselves.

The members of the various health professions and numerous health-oriented organizations cooperate in this educational effort, frequently by means of nationwide educational programs for the general public through the mass communication media or by local activities that reach more limited numbers of people. On an individual basis, the nursing practitioner has a unique contribution to make to the promotion of health because of frequent and close contact with people who are likely to be particularly conscious of their health at the time the nurse sees them. Through the function of teaching, applied at every appropriate opportunity, the nurse can help clients understand the importance of health principles and practices and help them assume the responsibility for applying what they learn to themselves and their families.

OPPORTUNITIES FOR TEACHING IN NURSING

Opportunities for the nurse to teach about health and illness are almost boundless; limitations arise only when the nurse fails to recognize situations favorable for teaching. If the practitioner does not see and use the opportunities at hand, all the teaching skill in the world and all the relevant knowledge about health will have no value.

Circumstances suitable for teaching may occur in a variety of nursing settings and with many different kinds of people. The range of such opportunities will be outlined in the following paragraphs. Clearly, no practitioner would ever have all these possibilities in one specific work setting, but since nurses may be employed in a number of different situations, they should be aware of the range of opportunities for teaching.

The practitioner will have opportunities to teach in any of the places where nursing service is given: in hospitals, clinics, and health situations; in homes; in schools; in industrial and business establishments; in doctors' offices.

The people the practitioner may teach include clients and co-workers. The clients have already been identified as the people to whom the nurse gives service, whether the service involves bedside care or health supervision. They are people of all ages, in all conditions of good health or illness, of various social and cultural backgrounds, and with all levels of education. They may be acutely ill or convalescent patients, the families of these patients, pregnant and postpartum women, school children and their parents, and employees in industry and business.

The practitioner's teaching may be needed by a great variety of co-workers. They include practical nurses, hospital nursing aides, public health nursing assistants, teachers and administrators in schools, supervisors in industry or business, medical clerks or secretaries, volunteer workers, and various community groups concerned with health problems. In certain circumstances, other nursing practitioners and students of nursing may also be taught. As with clients, co-workers may present great diversity in social, cultural, and educational backgrounds; they may also present wide variation in the extent of their knowledge and experience in relation to health and illness.

A BASIC PREMISE ABOUT THE PRACTITIONER'S TEACHING

After all this discussion about the variation among the people the nurse may teach and the situations in which teaching may take place, the question arises as to how the nurse can carry out the function of teaching among such divergent groups of people in so many different settings. There is one factor of similarity which is perhaps obvious, but which has great significance: all these learners are human beings and the basic processes of learning are the same for everyone, regardless of individual differences or variations in the teaching-learning situation. The practitioner who has a thorough understanding of the principles of teaching and learning and who knows how to apply them in nursing settings will find that the teaching function of the nurse is both a challenging and a satisfying responsibility.

A NOTE ABOUT REFERENCE READINGS IN *THIS* BOOK

The discussion in this book of the teaching function of the nursing practitioner involves many aspects of two professions—nursing and teaching. Because it is not possible to cover every area in detail, references to further reading are suggested at the end of each chapter. Since some of the readings do not relate specifically to nursing, the reader will, in some instances, have to make applications to the nursing setting.

REFERENCES

HIGHET, GILBERT. *The Art of Teaching.* New York: Vintage Books, 1954.
This classic book about teachers and teaching is recommended to the reader for its sound philosophy, its readability, and its delightful humor. It is an excellent introduction to the "art of teaching."

POHL, MARGARET L. "Teaching Activities of the Nursing Practitioner." *Nursing Research* 14:4-11, Winter, 1965.
This article summarizes a study of the teaching activities of nursing practitioners conducted by this author. The study served as a basis for the present book.

REDMAN, BARBARA K. "Patient Education as a Function of Nursing Practice." *Nursing Clinics of North America* 6:573-80, December, 1971.
The author agrees with the general philosophy of this book that teaching is an important function of nursing practice. In addition, the article points out some of the ways in which patient teaching might be improved.

Chapter _____ 2

Principles of Learning

Learning is an activity that is essential for the adequate development of the individual as an independent person and as a social being. It is the nature of human learning that is one of the characteristics that distinguishes us from other living creatures and makes possible what we know as human society.

Learning may be described as the process by which changes are brought about in an individual's response to his environment. His learning will depend upon the nature of his physical, mental, and emotional development and upon his past and present experiences. If we take into consideration the great variety of individual differences among human beings and the multiplicity of factors in the environment to which they are exposed, it becomes apparent that learning is never exactly the same for any two persons or, indeed, for any one person on different occasions.

Many studies have been done and many theories have been proposed to explain how learning occurs, what part is played by human capacities, and what part is played by environment. It is not our purpose here to weigh the pros and cons of educational theories, but rather to present some of the fundamental principles of learning to assist nursing practitioners in their efforts to teach people about health and illness.

DEFINITION OF PRINCIPLES

Principles are basic laws or truths that have been derived from man's past experience and that serve to explain the known facts in a particular area of knowledge. They may be modified upon further investigation, but in the meantime they represent that present wisdom; they serve as a guide for further investigation and give practical direction for present

6

action. Thus, physicists are continually conducting research to expand their knowledge of the scientific principles of the physical world, but in the meantime they base their explorations into outer space on the principles of physics that are already known. Psychologists continue to study human behavior to uncover deeper psychological truths, but at the same time they make practical applications of the psychological principles that are known today.

Some principles lie entirely within a specific field of knowledge. For example, the laws of heredity, concerning the transfer of the characteristics of parents to their offspring are principles in the realm of biology. Laws explaining the combination of elements into compounds are principles of chemistry. There are other principles, however, that have been derived from a combination of several areas of knowledge. The principles that explain how human beings behave are based on a synthesis of data from psychology, sociology, biology, chemistry, physics, and many other areas. It follows then, since learning is an aspect of human behavior, that the principles of learning are derived from the areas of knowledge that relate to the way people act and react in the great variety of situations to which they are exposed.

APPLICATION OF PRINCIPLES

It was stated above that principles serve as guides to action. It is not enough merely to know what principles are, or to be able to express a particular principle in words; it is also necessary to be able to apply these principles in actual situations. The nurse who understands and can recite the law of gravity has learned some theoretical physics; the nurse who applies this principle to the circulation of the blood and therefore elevates a patient's swollen leg to relieve the edema has made practical use of this knowledge for the benefit of the patient. In the same way, the nurse who understands the principles of learning must be able to make use of them in teaching, or the knowledge will be of no value to the patient.

In the following section of this chapter some of the basic principles of learning will be presented. An explanation of the principles will be given and will be followed by some examples to show how the practitioner might apply these principles in teaching in nursing situations.

PRINCIPLES OF LEARNING AND THEIR APPLICATIONS TO NURSING

Principle 1. Perception Is Necessary for Learning
Discussion

Perception is the process by which an individual becomes aware of his physical environment. Without this awareness learning is not possible.

Perception involves three steps: (1) the sense organs receive a stimulus; (2) the afferent nervous system transfers this impulse to a sensory area in the brain; and (3) the brain interprets it as a sensation of sight, sound, taste, odor, or touch. It is only through these pathways that we receive messages from the world around us.

Problems in perception occur because of individual differences among observers and because of actual errors in the way we perceive. Individual differences in the height of two persons, for example, can influence their perceptions: a grown man will perceive a particular dog as being rather small, while a child will perceive the same dog as being very large. As another example, the person who has always lived in the warm, humid climate of the tropics will perceive the climate of the temperate zone quite differently from the person who has always lived in northern latitudes.

Errors in perception are frequent. It is obvious that such errors will occur if the sensory apparatus is not functioning adequately, but many perceptual errors occur in individuals who have normal nervous systems. That we can easily have mistaken sensory impressions is demonstrated in popular books on optical illusions, by the sound-effects technicians of radio and television, and by the magician who can make us think we see things happen that do not in fact occur. Another cause of perceptual error is intense emotion, particularly fear. In the grip of emotion, the individual may perceive sensory stimuli incorrectly, or he may not be able to perceive them at all.

Regardless of the cause, individual differences in perception and unrecognized errors in perception constitute a serious problem in the process of learning.

Applications to Nursing

When a patient is admitted to a hospital for the first time, he is likely to be disturbed because of his illness. Adding to the stress is his exposure to many strange and often frightening stimuli. He must be given time to get his emotions under control and to experience this new environment with its unfamiliar sights and sounds and odors. The nurse must take the initiative in offering as much explanation as the patient may need and giving him a chance to ask questions about anything he does not understand. It is only by getting more experience and by receiving meaningful answers to his questions that he can correct his errors of perception. Since the nurse is in a familiar situation, it is easy to forget that this may not be the case for the patient. It would be helpful for the nurse to think back occasionally to the first day in the hospital as a student, to remember the feelings of confusion and insecurity, and to recall how important it was to have someone explain things and patiently answer questions. The nurse must be continually aware that unless an individual's perceptions are adequate, he cannot learn effectively.

The applications of this principle are especially important in attempting to teach patients who have any pathology in the sensory apparatus. If the sense receptors, the afferent nerves, or the sensory areas of the brain are damaged by disease or injury, certain perceptions will be impaired or, in some instances, completely lacking. There will be perceptual difficulties of varying degrees in patients who have impaired vision or hearing, in some patients with nerve or brain pathology, and, temporarily, with patients recovering from unconsciousness. The nurse must be aware of the possible extent of perceptual difficulty and modify teaching accordingly.

Principle 2.   Conditioning Is a Process of Learning
Discussion

Conditioning is the process by which a response that is aroused by a specific stimulus (A) can be aroused by an entirely different stimulus, (B) if the two stimuli are presented simultaneously over a sufficient length of time. A normal baby is born with a sucking reflex; he responds by sucking when a nipple is placed in his mouth (Stimulus A). If every time he is fed he sees a bottle (Stimulus B), he will eventually respond with the sucking reflex at the sight of the bottle without the nipple being placed in his mouth. As long as the sight of the bottle is followed immediately by feeding, the conditioned response will be reinforced—that is, strengthened. If, on the other hand, the sight of the bottle is *not* followed by feeding, the conditioned response will eventually be extinguished and the baby will no longer respond by sucking when he sees the bottle. This conditioning on a reflex level is one of the earliest and simplest forms of learning. Conditioning also occurs on a more complex level, as in the learning of habits and attitudes. It is probable that conditioning enters into all our learning to some extent.

It is important to realize that conditioning can be to our advantage or to our disadvantage. When we have been conditioned to the sound of an automobile horn so that our response is to look for an oncoming car when we hear a horn, this is to our advantage. When we have been conditioned as children to be suspicious of strangers, this may be to our disadvantage in later life when we want to make friends. The teacher who understands how conditioning occurs may be able to arrange learning experiences so that conditioned responses that are helpful to the learner can be reinforced and those that are detrimental can be extinguished.

Applications to Nursing

The practitioner's main concern with the learner's conditioned responses lies in the reinforcement of responses that are an asset to the learner and the extinction of responses that are or may become a liability. Suppose the nurse is caring for a small child who has learned the habit of feeding himself at home. The nurse may reinforce the habit by arranging his tray at mealtime so he can feed himself, by showing approval of any attempt he makes to feed himself, and by alerting the others who give him care to do the same. This is particularly important for the child who is going to have to stay in the hospital for an extended period; if he is fed regularly by the nursing staff for some time, he may become conditioned to being fed and may lose the independence he had previously attained.

Frequently the nurse will care for a child who has been conditioned to fear doctors and nurses or, to be more exact, to fear people wearing white uniforms. He has learned to associate white clothing with being sick, painful injections, or bad-tasting medicine. Trying to reason with this youngster will not change his response; the nurse can help him to develop pleasant associations with doctors and nurses by being gentle, talking quietly and playing with him, and, when painful procedures must be done, by explaining to him what is going to be done and by telling him honestly that it will hurt, if this is the case. Any confidence you may have built up in him in relation to doctors and nurses will be completely shattered if you lie to him when he asks "Is it going to hurt?"

Changing this attitude of fear about doctors and nurses is important, not only for the child's present hospital stay, but also, perhaps, for the future. Adults who have been negatively conditioned in this way in their childhood, very often tend to avoid doctors and nurses except in dire emergency. Often the emergency could have been avoided rather easily if they had had regular physical examinations or had come for help when they first became ill.

Principle 3. The Process of Trial-and-Error
Is a Way of Learning

Discussion

When we are faced with a situation to which we do not know how to respond, we may refuse to react by retreating from the situation if that is possible or, if we must act, we make random hit-or-miss responses. If the situation is not beyond our capacities, this random behavior will sooner or later produce a response which seems appropriate. This success reinforces the response, we repeat it, and by further practice we learn this particular response to this situation. This is called trial-and-error learning. We see it in the behavior of a person who wants to solve a mechanical puzzle but has no idea of how to go about it. He moves the pieces of the puzzle in many chance ways until he happens to make the motion that unlocks it. He may not realize at the moment just what he did to solve the puzzle, so he goes through the random motions again until he discovers which move was successful. He thus learns to solve the puzzle. We sometimes also use trial-and-error in attempting to solve purely intellectual problems.

It is obvious that trial-and-error learning is wasteful in terms of time and energy spent and the great number of incorrect trials that may have to be made before the correct response is learned. However, if we have had no relevant experience of our own and do not have the benefit of someone else's experience, trial-and-error is our only recourse in new situations. This fact points up an important function of the teacher, which is to guide the learner toward the correct response and help him avoid at least some ineffective activity, even though the learner will still have to use the trial-and-error approach to learn the correct responses for himself. For example, in learning to ride a bicycle the learner must use some trial-and-error behavior, but a teacher may be able to make some suggestions that will eliminate many unsuccessful trials and help the learner accomplish his goal more efficiently.

Applications to Nursing

The nurse will often have occasion to teach patients, family members, and co-workers how to perform treatments that require certain physical dexterity in handling equipment. Demonstrating for the learner what is to be done is the logical first step, but it must be followed by giving him an opportunity to become familiar with the equipment and to practice using it. The nurse must expect the learner to make mistakes at first since this is to a certain extent trial-and-error learning, but if the nurse takes the errors as a matter of course and calmly suggests how to correct them, the learner will more quickly master the skill than if he is left to his own devices. The nurse's approval and encouragement will also help to reinforce the learning.

Principle 4. Learning May Occur Through Imitation
Discussion

Imitation plays an important part in learning. Sometimes the process is unconscious, as when we "pick up" the mannerisms, vocabulary, or attitudes of the people with whom we associate; sometimes we imitate consciously, as when someone shows us how to do something and we attempt to copy what we have observed. The ability to imitate depends on the skills the learner has already acquired. If he is to imitate speech patterns, he must have already learned to control his speech mechanisms;

if he is to imitate a manual skill, he must already have the necessary control of his hands and arms.

Teachers can make good use, in many ways, of the learner's ability to imitate, but it is important to remember that the learner may be imitating things in the teacher's behavior that were not planned as part of the learning experience as, for example, personal mannerisms, incorrect speech, or negative attitudes. The teacher, by virtue of the fact that there is a certain status and authority inherent in teaching, is setting an example constantly. It is the teacher's responsibility to see to it, as far as possible, that the learner is imitating desirable behavior.

Applications to Nursing

The demonstration method of teaching is often used in nursing. It is clear that this way of teaching makes use of the learner's ability to imitate. The nurse must be sure that the learner is physically able to perform the necessary actions and must allow sufficient repetition and practice for the learner to master the technique, since trial-and-error learning is usually involved in learning by imitation.

Since the learner may imitate whatever he sees, the nurse who is functioning as a teacher of health must consistently demonstrate good health practices. The nurse who is well groomed, who comes to work having had enough sleep, who is obviously in good health, is in a position to teach health concepts by example. When the nurse does not exemplify good health habits, the patient's reaction may well be, "What you *do* speaks so loudly that I cannot hear what you are saying."

Principle 5. The Development of Concepts Is Part of the Learning Process
Discussion

A concept is a meaningful idea or mental picture that an individual holds. Concepts may relate to inanimate objects, natural forces, people, events, ideas—in fact, we develop concepts about anything we can think about. Since conceptualization is a process that occurs entirely within the learner's mind, it is the learner who must develop the concepts. The teacher can help by understanding the process in order to give assistance when it is needed. The teacher can also help by making sure that the concepts the learner develops are valid, by asking questions, and by having the learner explain the concept in words.

Conceptualization is a complex process involving six components: (1) perceptions, (2) emotions, (3) verbal symbols or words, (4) integration, (5) generalization, and (6) abstraction. The process may occur on both the conscious and unconscious levels. As an example, we will trace the development of a relatively simple concept, the concept of "dog."

When the young child sees a dog for the first time, he gets sensory impressions (perceptions) of the physical appearance and behavior of the dog. As his experience with a variety of dogs increases, his perceptions increase. He sees dogs of different sizes, shapes, colors, and different ways of behaving. At the same time, he may develop emotional reactions, either pleasant or unpleasant, depending on his experience. These feelings are the basis for his future attitude about dogs and form part of his concept of "dog."

Sooner or later, the child learns verbal symbols that help him develop his concept further. He learns the word "dog" and realizes that this sound represents a dog. As his vocabulary increases and he understands descriptive words like *big, little, black, brown,* he can begin to make comparisons among the dogs he sees, and express similarities and differences. He becomes aware that dogs in general have four legs, a head, and a tail, and they can bark; he also notices that dogs are of different colors, sizes, and dispositions. As he observes other animals, he sees that cats and horses also have four legs, a head, and a tail, but they are different from dogs and they have a different relationship to him: he pets a cat, he rides a horse, he throws a ball for the dog to fetch. This process of understanding similarities, differences, and functional relationships is called *integration.*

The next step in conceptualization is *generalization.* The child learns that all dogs have certain common characteristics; now when he sees a dog he has never seen before, he can classify it as a dog. He has generalized his concept of "dog" to include all dogs.

The last step is *abstraction.* The child learns to understand what qualities constitute "dog-ness" and he can handle the idea of "dog" without making reference to any particular dog. At this point he has a well-developed concept of "dog," but the concept will continue to be modified and broadened with further experience with dogs.

This discussion illustrates the development of a comparatively simple concept. With wider experience and greater ability to integrate, generalize, and make abstractions in the realm of ideas, the individual is able to master increasingly complex relationships; for example, the development of scientific principles, philosophical values, or advanced theories in any area of knowledge all depend on highly abstract conceptualization.

In summary, then, concepts are built up through a sequence of processes or steps. Clearly, with all these interdependent components, individuals may frequently make errors in developing their concepts. It is important to remember that we develop our concepts within our own minds and we take for granted that they are correct, unless they are proven to be not valid either through our own added experience or the help of someone else. An important aspect of both teaching and learning is the correction of *mis*conceptions through reeducation.

Applications to Nursing

By the time that most individuals are old enough to be concerned with learning concepts about health and illness, they have had practice in developing their skills of conceptualization; their vocabulary has increased greatly; and they have had a good deal of experience in integrating, generalizing, and working out abstractions. It is true that they will probably also have some misconceptions that will have to be corrected, but they have developed far beyond the level of the child who is learning the concept of "dog." Thus, the practitioner will be able to some extent to draw upon the learner's mental skills and experience in conceptualization in presenting new concepts that he needs to know. The nurse's role consists in supplying the information he needs to know to develop the concept, in clarifying his ideas, and in evaluating the validity of the final concept. Sometimes the nurse must also help to resolve emotional attitudes that may be interfering with learning.

Let us suppose that the nurse is caring for a patient who has had severe burns on his chest and arms. He has been in the hospital for several days and healing is progressing without any complications, but the nurse notices that he lies almost motionless in bed and is completely dependent on the nursing personnel for his care. It is clear that this patient must move about in bed as much as possible and begin to help care for himself to prevent physical complications such as contractures, pneumonia, embolus formation, and decubitus ulcers, and also the psychological effects of prolonged dependence. It may not be enough merely to tell the patient he must exercise, since he may simply refuse to exercise or exercise only when the nurse is in the room. For him to understand the need for activity, he must develop a concept of the relation of self-help to his eventual recovery and independence. Let it be said here, however, that it is not necessary or advisable to point out in graphic detail all the possible complications which might result from inactivity; our purpose is to encourage the patient to exercise, not to immobilize him further by fear.

The first step in working with this particular patient is to find out why his activity has become so limited. The fact that he remains almost motionless, although there is no physical reason why he cannot move to some extent, is a cue that there may be an emotional factor or a misconception that prevents him from behaving as he normally would. By suggesting that he make some specific motion, such as turning over or moving himself up in bed, the nurse opens the way for him to express what the problem is: perhaps he thought he was supposed to lie still, perhaps it is painful to move, perhaps he is afraid he will cause damage to the burns. Whatever the problem is, the patient must be given the opportunity to talk about it and the nurse must accept the thoughts and feelings he expresses. No matter how naïve or unreal the patient's ideas may appear to the nurse, this is what the patient believes and this is where the nurse must start in order to help him correct errors and resolve emotional conflicts.

During this interchange, the nurse may discover what the patient already knows about the importance of exercise in normal daily living. By giving him information that will help him to understand the relation of exercise to his present illness and the importance of self-help in reestablishing his independence, the nurse may facilitate the patient's development of these concepts which are so essential for his return to normal health and activity. Finally, the nurse can test the validity of his concepts by encouraging the patient to talk about them and by observing how effectively he actually applies them. If he continues to be dependent and makes no effort to move about in bed, or if, on the other hand, he exerts himself too much, the nurse must reevaluate the situation to find out what is wrong. Whether the problem lies with the teacher or the learner is irrelevant; it is the nurse's responsibility to discover what the problem is, and correct it, if possible.

Principle 6. An Individual Must Be Motivated in Order to Learn
Discussion

Motivation is a force or drive within an individual which makes him take action. This state may be aroused by a physical need, an emotion, or an idea, but whatever the cause, motivation always stimulates the individual to *do* something. We are being motivated by physical needs when hunger makes us move toward food or when pain makes us move away from an uncomfortable stimulus. When emotions motivate us, we may move toward or away from a situation, depending on the nature of the emotions that have been aroused. Ideas may serve as motivating forces; they may produce simple and immediate results or highly complex activities which go on over a long period of time. For instance, the idea that dinner is nearly ready may lead us to go to wash our hands; the idea that we want to enter a professional field at some time in the distant future may lead us to devote many years of concentrated effort in the direction of that goal.

From these examples, it should be clear that motivation may be a fleeting impulse or a prolonged, sustained force. For the individual to be moved in the direction of learning, the motivation must persist throughout the learning process. It is important to be aware, however, that motivation takes place within the individual; it cannot be superimposed by someone else. It is possible to treat the learner in ways that will encourage him to want to learn; it is possible to present material to be learned in ways that will make learning easier; but the fact remains that the learner himself must develop the motivation for learning.

Another aspect of motivation must be understood before it is possible to help people develop motivation to learn. The potential learner's motivation will automatically be directed toward his most pressing need at the moment. If his physical needs are dominant, he will be motivated toward relieving these stresses; if his emotions have the upper hand, he will try to get relief from these pressures. He can only be motivated to learn when the desire to learn is stronger than his other drives. Even when he wants to learn, his energies may suddenly be redirected into different channels when other needs become dominant. All of us have experienced this phenomenon at some time during our schooling. We were motivated to study an assignment and settled down to work, only to be diverted, against our wishes, by some pressing family matter. It is important to be aware that this redirection of attention and motivation because of a need that takes precedence over all others is beyond the control of the individual. When these other more pressing problems have been resolved, the individual will be able to direct his attention again to the learning process.

Applications to Nursing

Whether the potential learners in nursing situations are clients or co-workers, sick or well, they must be motivated if they are to learn. If they already want to learn, perhaps because of natural curiosity, or because they understand the importance of good health, or because they have experienced illness and want to get well and stay well, they are, by definition, already motivated and the nurse will have few problems in this area. On the other hand, if they show no interest in learning, the nurse will face a real challenge in trying to discover the reason for their indifference and in attempting to overcome it.

There is no simple formula that can be applied to stimulate people to want to learn. The practitioner must get to know each learner and assess the reason for lack of interest. With patients, the cause is often the pressures of their illness or their emotional state; in such cases, teaching will have to be delayed until the illness or the emotional stress has been alleviated. Another common problem is that the potential learner sees no reason for learning what the nurse wants to teach him. Here the nurse will have to help the learner see the need by appealing to his desire to get well or stay well or, in the case of parents, their desire to maintain their children's good health.

Sometimes co-workers, for example nursing assistants, are apathetic because they feel there is no point in trying to learn more in order to improve their work, since no one cares or will notice if they do; they may feel that they will always be called to task for their errors, but never get credit for doing good work. This attitude is sometimes justified; under the pressures of work on a busy nursing unit, we have to find time to correct errors, but we do not always take time to give praise for a job well done. If the worker receives recognition for good work, he may feel encouraged to improve his performance and thus be motivated to learn.

These are but a few examples of how the practitioner can encourage motivation to learn. As we have said, it is the learner who has to develop the motivation. If the nurse has done as much as possible to stimulate motivation without producing any apparent effect, there may be a deeper problem which will require the kind of help that the nurse is not equipped to give. It is just as important to realize that a situation is beyond our capabilities as it is to recognize situations that we can handle. In most cases, however, the nurse who gets to know the client or co-worker and applies the principles of learning and teaching to the particular situation at hand will be able to help him to develop motivation for learning.

Principle 7. Physical and Mental Readiness Are Necessary for Learning

Discussion

Readiness for learning refers to the learner's ability to learn in terms of his physical and mental development. It is not related to whether an individual *wants* to learn (which is his motivation), but rather to whether he is *able* to learn at a given time in his life. Physical readiness depends primarily on the state of the individual's neuromuscular system and is chiefly relevant to learning physical skills. Observation of normal infants will show that there is a definite progression of physical abilities which appear as the child's muscles and nerve pathways develop: holding his head erect, sitting without support, crawling, walking; the child cannot perform these skills until his musculature is strong enough to provide support and his nervous system well-developed enough to coordinate these complex activities. Mental readiness depends on the state of the individual's intellectual development. He must, of course, have enough intellectual capacity for the learning task, but in addition, he must have had adequate experience in the perceptions, verbalizations, and concept formation which he needs for further learning.

The teacher must attempt to distinguish between lack of readiness and lack of motivation, because these problems must be handled differently. We have already discussed some of the ways of encouraging motivation. When the problem is clearly one of inability to learn because of the state of the individual's development, he must be given the time and opportunity for normal growth and maturation or the subject matter must be adapted to the level he has reached.

Applications to Nursing

The practitioner must be aware of the importance of readiness in teaching all kinds of learners. There are certain patients, however, who merit the nurse's particular attention in this connection. These are the patients who, although they have reached physical and intellectual maturation, have now developed disease or suffered injury affecting their neuromuscular systems; for example, patients who have had a cerebrovascular accident or extensive trauma to muscles. These patients must go through a healing process before function can be resumed; often reeducation will be necessary. Whether it is learning to walk again, or to speak, or to think, reeducation is impossible until the patient has regained the necessary physical or mental ability and is ready for learning. If the nurse understands this concept in relation to these patients, it will be possible to give the patient the encouragement he will need in his attempts to relearn things which he knows "any child can do." If the patient's condition is such that he is either temporarily or permanently unable to learn, the nurse will have to teach those who will be responsible for the patient's welfare when he leaves the hospital.

Principle 8. Effective Learning Requires Active Participation

Discussion

If an individual is to learn, he must become actively involved in the learning process. Simply stated, he learns by doing, and the "doing" may involve a variety of activities: perceiving through the sense organs, carrying out physical actions, or using mental processes. This involvement is essential for learning and the more thoroughly the individual participates, the more effective will be the learning which results.

Consider, for example, a piano student who is learning a new composition. How does he become involved actively? He listens to the teacher play the piece, he makes mental or written notes of the teacher's suggestions; he uses his eyes to read the musical notes and his eyes and hands to find the corresponding keys on the piano; he counts the meter out loud or in his mind; he notices how his hands feel when the right chords are played; he practices the piece time and again, listening to how it sounds; he begins to memorize the notes; with further practice he becomes more skillful in technique and expression, he recalls more readily what he has already partially memorized and recognizes phrases that are repeated in the composition; finally, he "knows it by heart," and can play it with good technique and expression. He has learned the piece. His senses, his physical actions, and his mental processes have all been called into play. His active participation has made effective learning possible.

This example is concerned with learning a skill. The same principle of learning by doing applies to all learning, whether it is learning skills, facts, principles, ideas: the more the learner participates, the more likely he is to learn well and to remember what he has learned.

Applications to Nursing

The need for active participation for effective learning applies to all nursing situations; the function of the nurse is to provide opportunities for participation and to encourage the learner to take advantage of them. For example, the practitioner who is teaching a nursing assistant about the care of a particular patient may begin by having him watch the nurse give the care, by giving him the written procedure to read, and by encouraging him to ask questions. As he becomes familiar with what is involved, he may begin to assist in giving the care, later discussing any problems he has. When the nurse is assured that there is no question of the patient's safety, the assistant may carry out the procedure himself and evaluate his performance with the nurse's help. With further practice under less close supervision by the nurse, he will develop the skill and the confidence he needs to administer the care he has been learning to give. He will have learned through active participation.

Principle 9. New Learning Must Be Based on Previous Knowledge and Experience

Discussion

Learning is an evolving process in which each step must be mastered before the next step can be learned. We cannot learn to spell until we know the letters of the alphabet; we cannot learn arithmetic until we have some concept of numbers; we cannot learn a complex skill until we have mastered the simpler skills involved. You can probably recall an occasion when you were absent from school for a time and returned to find your classmates studying subject matter which you could not understand; you had missed some of the "previous knowledge" necessary for understanding the new material, and you had to go back and learn what you had missed in order to catch up with the class.

This principle is applied in the organization of the courses in an educational program. The subjects are planned in a sequence that requires the completion of basic courses before advanced courses may be taken;

elementary algebra is a prerequisite for intermediate algebra, and general chemistry precedes advanced chemistry.

When an individual is unable to learn what is being taught, it may have little to do with his intellectual capacity; perhaps he does not have the prerequisite knowledge or experience that he needs in order to master the present learning task.

Applications to Nursing

The principle we have just discussed is not a difficult one to understand, but the nurse must be sure not only to understand it but to apply it. Planning for teaching a particular topic should include consideration of what prior knowledge and experience are necessary for an understanding of the subject and should provide for specific ways of determining whether the learner has that knowledge. If the nurse, for example, intends to teach a patient about the therapeutic diet prescribed for him by the doctor, it is important to find out what he already knows about normal nutrition and perhaps his knowledge of how his illness affects his body's ability to utilize various foods. This can usually be accomplished best by introducing the subject and then encouraging the patient to talk about what he already knows by asking him some general questions. Many patients will respond to rather specific questions and some will volunteer information. The point at which the nurse begins teaching will be determined by the extent of the learner's knowledge and experience about nutrition and diet.

It is important to keep in mind the purpose for which the teaching is being done—in this case, to insure that the patient will follow his diet. Keeping the objective in focus will help the nurse to limit the teaching to the essentials and not try to teach, more than the patient needs to know. If it becomes clear that the patient is interested in learning more than this, the nurse might give him material to read. The time that is available for teaching must be used for the essentials necessary to accomplish nursing goals since the practitioner has many other duties besides teaching.

Principle 10. The Emotional Climate Affects Learning
Discussion

We have already discussed the influence of emotions on sensory perception, in the development of concepts and in motivation; we have pointed out that a strong negative emotion, such as fear, can prevent rational behavior. Intense positive feelings, like great joy or the feeling of relief when a crisis is safely passed, can also dominate our reactions.

In the same way, strong emotions can influence learning behavior. It may be argued that a person who is in a panic of fear that he will not pass an important examination may study very hard and pass in spite of his emotions. This may be true, but there are several other facts about this situation that may also be true: the individual's motivation for passing the test was strong enough so that he could control his fear to some extent; he might have learned the material better if he had not been afraid; and it is likely that he merely memorized and may forget most of what he has "learned" as soon as the test is over. In other words, even in this apparently successful effort, fear probably prevented optimum learning.

In general it may be said that if the emotional climate is neutral or just positive or negative enough to produce motivation, effective learning may be possible; if the emotional climate is extreme, little if any effective learning can take place.

Applications to Nursing

Emotional overtones are likely to be present in many nursing situations. Think of the possibilities from the point of view of the patient in the hospital: the fact of his illness with its pain, discomfort, and debilitating effects; the strangeness of the hospital setting; the removal from his family and his normal habits of living; the worry of unemployment for the wage earner and the worry about the children's welfare for the parent; the multitude of other worries and fears to which all human beings are subject; and, in many cases, the fear of permanent disability or of death. The patient's family is also suffering many of these fears along with the patient, and must also make readjustments caused by the patient's absence from the family group.

Many of the same fears are present when the patient is ill at home. In addition, while the fear of strange surroundings is not present, the very fact that the patient is at home and incapacitated may be disruptive both for him and for his family, and the family has the additional problem of adjusting to his illness and of taking responsibility for his care.

The nurse's co-workers in the hospital may also be subject to emotional strains not characteristic of workers in most other kinds of employment. Responsibility for the welfare and safety of their patients, reactions to the crises which so often develop in hospitals, involvement in the patient's problems and worries—all these factors may be added to complicate the usual stresses of daily life.

The practitioner may be able to help the patient, the family member, or the co-worker to handle these emotions by encouraging him to talk about them; "just talking" to a receptive listener may relieve some of the tension and may also help to clarify the problem. However, just letting someone who is upset talk may prove to be more destructive than helpful if the nurse makes the mistake of contradicting what he says or denying the reality of his fears or offering such platitudes as "Everything will be all right," or "You really shouldn't worry." The person who is worried has a reason for worrying and until he is able to explore these feelings, he cannot begin to handle them, nor can anyone help him. If he receives responses from the nurse which tend to cut off his expression of his feelings, he will either be more disturbed because he can see that the nurse does not understand, or he will thereafter conceal his feelings and thus be further than ever from resolving his problems.

Sometimes we err in the opposite direction. We assume that because a particular situation would make us feel a certain way, it would necessarily make someone else feel the same way and for the same reason. An example of an actual incident will perhaps make the point clear. The mother of a growing family was admitted to the hospital for surgery for a brain tumor. Prior to the operation it was obvious that she was very much disturbed, but she refused to talk about what was bothering her. The nursing staff "naturally" assumed she was worried about the outcome of the surgery and whether her husband and children were all right. They tried to reassure her about the surgery, and, after contacting her husband, told her that everything was going well at home; their efforts were of no avail. Finally someone on the staff was able to get the patient to talk and discovered that, although she was concerned about the operation and about her family, that was not the major emotional problem for her. She knew her head had to be shaved before surgery and all she could think of was, "How can I face my family and my friends without my hair?" The idea of wearing a turban or a wig until her hair grew out had not occurred to her; all she could visualize was her shaved head. Obviously not all emotional problems can be handled as easily as this one; the point here is that the nurse must find out what is really bothering the individual, and not make assumptions on the basis of what the nurse thinks is causing the difficulty.

Principle 11. Repetition Strengthens Learning
   Discussion

A large part of learning occurs through the formation of habits of one kind or another. Habits are well-established patterns of behavior which can be developed only through practice and repetition. Different learners need varying amounts of repetition for effective learning, but all learners need a certain amount of it. In addition, habits tend to weaken when they are not used frequently after they have been learned. Thus, repetition is essential to maintain habits. Perhaps you studied a foreign language in high school. You can remember how much practice and repetition you needed to master grammar, vocabulary, and pronunciation.

If you have had occasion to use that language regularly, you may be quite proficient in it by now. If, on the other hand, you have not spoken, read, or listened to that tongue since the day you stopped studying it, you are well aware of how lack of use can weaken or even extinguish a habit.

Applications to Nursing

People who are learning about health and illness need practice and repetition for adequate learning just as they do in other subject matter. The hospital nurse today faces a problem in this respect because of the patient's shortened hospitalization which sometimes does not allow enough time for the practice and repetition necessary for really thorough learning. In some situations, not a great deal can be done about this, but if the patient is to be referred to a clinic or to a public health nursing agency, provision can be made for the hospital nurse to report on the referral form what teaching has been started so that the nurse who will take over the care or supervision of the patient after discharge can continue from the point where the hospital nurse left off.

Principle 12. Satisfaction Reinforces Learning
Discussion

The fact that satisfaction reinforces learning is bound up closely with the concept of motivation. We tend to want to do again the things that we enjoy doing. Sometimes we get satisfaction from learning entirely from within ourselves: because of a feeling of accomplishment, because our curiosity about something has been satisfied, because we see how the learning benefits us, because the learning experience was a pleasant one. We may also feel rewarded by external factors, such as approval and encouragement from people whose opinions we value. No matter what the source, satisfaction reinforces our learning in the present situation and also tends to make us want to learn more.

It should be mentioned here that moderate amounts of dissatisfaction can also stimulate learning. Doing poorly on a test on which we feel we could have done better, or not being able to perform some skill as well as we would like to, can serve to make us put forth more effort and thus learn better. However, if failure is too great or occurs too consistently, the result very often will be to discourage any further attempts to try to succeed in the area where we have experienced so much failure. The teacher can sometimes counteract this feeling of failure by providing easier learning situations in which the learner can succeed and thus help him to regain the feeling of satisfaction he needs in order to continue to learn.

Applications to Nursing

The nurse can stimulate feelings of satisfaction in learning situations by establishing a pleasant atmosphere, by helping the learner see how the learning will benefit him, by giving approval and encouragement, and, if the learner shows signs of becoming discouraged, by simplifying the subject matter if possible, or presenting a learning task at which he is sure to succeed.

Making consistent efforts to provide satisfaction in learning is particularly important in teaching clients, because in nursing situations clients are not required to learn as they are in school or in work settings. Clients may be said to be "voluntary learners" and many times one of the greatest challenges to the practitioner is to get the client to want to learn. Providing satisfaction is one way to stimulate motivation to learn.

SUMMARY

The material presented in this chapter is summarized here by restating the principles of learning which have been discussed.
1. Perception is necessary for learning.
2. Conditioning is a process of learning.
3. The process of trial-and-error is a way of learning.
4. Learning may occur through imitation.
5. The development of concepts is part of the learning process.
6. An individual must be motivated in order to learn.
7. Physical and mental readiness are necessary for learning.
8. Effective learning requires active participation.
9. New learning must be based on previous knowledge and experience.
10. The emotional climate affects learning.
11. Repetition strengthens learning.
12. Satisfaction reinforces learning.

For additional material on these principles, it is suggested that the reader refer to basic psychology textbooks and the annotated references listed below.

REFERENCES

AIKEN, LINDA HARMAN. "Patient Problems Are Problems in Learning." *American Journal of Nursing* 70:1916-18, September, 1970.
This author maintains that it is not enough to "do teaching"; nurses must help patients cope with their environment more effectively after evaluating each patient's abilities and his need for help.
BARNARD, MILDRED E. "Toward the Development of Sound Health Concepts." *Nursing Outlook* 10:406-8, June, 1962.

The author discusses the need for sound health concepts as a basis for good health practices, and emphasizes the nurse's role in helping the learner to develop or modify his concepts.

BERNARD, HAROLD M. *Psychology of Learning and Teaching*, 2d ed. New York: McGraw-Hill Book Company, 1965.
This book contains excellent material relevant to learning in nursing settings. The chapters on habit formation, factors facilitating learning, and the emotional aspects of learning will be of particular value.

CARNEVALI, DORIS L. "Preoperative Anxiety." *American Journal of Nursing* 66:1536-38, July, 1966.
This discussion of preoperative anxiety and the difficulties of identifying its underlying causes is relevant in assessing the emotional climate of learning situations.

GOULD, GRACE THERESA, ed. "Symposium on Compassion and Communication in Nursing." *Nursing Clinics of North America* 4:651-729, December, 1969.
The articles of this symposium make clear the essential role of empathy and compassion as part of effective nurse-patient and teacher-learner communication.

JOHNSON, BETTY SUE. "The Meaning of Touch in Nursing." *Nursing Outlook* 13:59-60, February, 1965.
The author discusses the sense of touch in relation to nursing and suggests some factors that determine how both nurses and patients may react to this important avenue of perception.

KENDLER, HOWARD H. *Basic Psychology*, 2d ed. New York: Appleton-Century-Crofts, 1968.
This basic text is well illustrated and emphasizes psychological research. Sections particularly appropriate for the practitioner are those dealing with perception, learning and forgetting, and frustration and conflict.

REDMAN, BARBARA K. "Readiness for Health Education," in *The Process of Patient Teaching in Nursing*. St. Louis: C. V. Mosby, 1968, pp. 15-39.
The author has included interesting and valuable material on health beliefs and behaviors, motivating factors, and a section on assessing patient readiness for learning.

UJHELY, GERTRUD B. *Determinants of the Nurse-Patient Relationship*. New York: Springer, 1968.
This entire book is relevant to the teacher-learner relationship in nursing, but the reader's attention is called particularly to "Part III. What the Patient Brings to the Relationship."

WU, RUTH. "Explaining Treatments to Young Children." *American Journal of Nursing* 65:71-73, July, 1965.
The processes of concept formation, generalization, and abstraction are clearly presented in this discussion of how nurses can explain treatments to the 2- to 8-year-old child.

Chapter _____ 3

Principles of Teaching

Teaching is the art of helping people to learn. The teacher can facilitate learning not only by means of a thorough understanding of the learning process, but also by developing specific skills and abilities in teaching. It would be very convenient if it were possible to set up a list of rules for teaching that could be followed step by step in order to guarantee effective teaching. However, the many human and environmental variables that may influence the teaching-learning process make it impossible to set up formulas for teaching; each learner is unique and each learning situation is different. Successful teaching is facilitated by a knowledge of the principles of teaching and the ability to apply them to specific situations.

THE SOURCE OF TEACHING PRINCIPLES

The principles of teaching are derived from the principles of learning; what the teacher does is determined either directly or indirectly by the way people learn. For example, we have pointed out that people learn by taking an active part in the teaching-learning process, therefore the teacher plans activities for the learner; imitation is a way of learning, therefore the teacher attempts to set a good example for the learner; repetition is necessary for learning, therefore the teacher allows time for this in planning for teaching. Thus, the teacher is guided both generally and in specific situations by understanding and being able to apply the principles of learning. As the principles of teaching are being presented in this chapter, it is important to keep in mind the learning principles that have already been discussed in order to see how each suggestion for teaching depends on some aspect of the learning process. This chapter will serve as an introduction to the more detailed consideration of various aspects of teaching that will be presented in later chapters.

PRINCIPLES OF TEACHING IN NURSING SETTINGS

Principle 1. Good Nurse-Learner Rapport Is Important in Teaching

The ability to establish a comfortable relationship or rapport with another person is important in any kind of cooperative effort, and co-operation enhances the teaching-learning process. The nurse may be aware of the need of the client or co-worker to learn and may be eager to teach him, but it is the learner who must do the learning. By establishing a positive, constructive relationship with the learner, the nurse will have taken the first step toward bringing about a climate that will encourage the learner's cooperation. Good rapport will not of itself guarantee successful teaching, but it is a condition that facilitates teaching and is a factor that the nurse can control to a large extent.

Establishing a good teacher-learner relationship also makes it possible to get to know the learner as a person so that the nurse can assess to some extent those elements that determine how effective teaching will be: the learner's previous knowledge and experience, his readiness for learning, his motivation. The nurse may also begin to get an idea of what teaching is needed in relation to health concepts.

In an earlier chapter we discussed the fact that many people (including patients and their families) react negatively to nurses because of previous experiences. Many people also have the same kind of reaction to teachers. When you are identified by the learner as both a nurse and a teacher, you may be subject to such responses through no fault of your own. It is impossible to overcome such feelings merely by talking; the most effective way to modify your learner's opinion of nurses and teachers is by your own behavior. A positive "living example" is a very effective teaching tool. It is not *necessary* for the learner to like the teacher, but it certainly helps. This is especially true of the nurse-client relationship where the learner is free to remove himself either physically or mentally from the learning situation if he chooses to do so.

Rapport is as important to the learner as to the teacher. If the learner is to be able to ask the questions and make the mistakes that are a part of the process of learning, he must feel comfortable with the nurse. He will take the teaching more seriously if he has respect for the nurse as a person and a practitioner, and feels that the example the nurse sets is worth imitating. If he sees evidence that the nurse is really interested in teaching him and is genuinely concerned for his welfare, his motivation for learning will probably be strengthened.

Good teacher-learner relationships are established in the same way that the nurse establishes good relationships with patients. The reader, whether you are a student of nursing or a graduate nurse practitioner, already knows a good deal about establishing rapport. Our purpose here is to review briefly some of the principles involved to see how they can be applied in nursing settings to develop an atmosphere that will be conducive to learning.

Our general approach to the people we want to teach has a marked effect on the relationships we establish. Each learner is a unique human being, worthy of our respect and having the same rights to which all human beings are entitled. As nurses, we probably subscribe to this belief, but there are many times when we fail to *act* on it and, as often as not, we are not fully aware of why this happens.

One of the reasons we may have difficulty in seeing each person as a unique individual is because of the way human beings think. There are so many discrete things in the world around us that we must be able to classify them and generalize about them as groups in order to be able to think clearly about them. The trouble arises when we put unlike things into the same classification or make errors in identifying the common characteristics of that class.

When we discussed the process of concept formation, we spoke about generalization, and cited as an example that when a child learns that all dogs have certain common characteristics, he can classify a new dog as a dog and thus has generalized his concept of "dog" to include all dogs. This is an essential step in learning about our environment. But suppose the child makes an error and classifies a rabbit as a dog; he will be surprised that the rabbit does not behave as he expects it to on the basis of his experience with dogs. Suppose he has generalized that all dogs are friendly, since all the dogs he has seen were friendly; he will certainly run into trouble if he acts on this assumption and tries to play with an unfriendly dog.

We tend to do the same thing with people. We classify them into groups and build up a picture; then we assume that these characteristics are qualities of anyone whom we classify as a member of a particular group. These "models" that we develop are called *stereotypes*, a word taken from the printing industry where a mold, called a stereotype, is cast and then used to produce hundreds of identical copies of printed materials. Usually the less we know about a group of people, the more rigid and inaccurate our stereotype is. If, for example, we have known *just one* Irish family and all the members were red-haired, blue-eyed, and quick-tempered, we may expect that anyone who is Irish has these characteristics or, on the other hand, that any red-haired, blue-eyed, quick-tempered person must be Irish. If it strikes you that no graduate nurse or student of nursing could ever develop such a stereotype, that may be because you have known *many* red-haired, blue-eyed, quick-tempered people who were not Irish, and *many* Irish people who did not have red hair, blue eyes, and quick tempers. Remember, we said stereotypes are developed on the basis of little or no actual experience with the people we are stereotyping.

We have emphasized stereotypes here because they are such a common mechanism and because stereotypes completely negate the uniqueness and individuality of the person involved. It is so easy to conclude, "There now, I've classified him; I know what the people in his group are like; I know what he is like." It takes much more effort, after you have classified him, to take the next step: "How is he different from most of the people I know in this group? In what ways is he unlike *anyone* else?" In other words, "What is this person like, how does he behave and why, what does he feel and think about things?" Clearly, we cannot answer all these questions about any of our learners, but we can make an attempt to really view them as individuals, not stereotypes. Our stereotypes may be complimentary or detrimental or neutral; in any case, they serve to prevent us from establishing valid relationships because they prevent us from getting to know our learner as a person.

Another block to good interpersonal relationships is our prejudices. A prejudice is a pre-judgment; it implies that we come to conclusions without sufficient evidence to support our judgments. We may learn our prejudices from the people with whom we have associated throughout our lives, as is made so clear in the line, "You've got to be taught to hate," from a song in the Broadway show "South Pacific." Or we may develop our prejudices ourselves in the course of our own limited experience. It is very difficult to free ourselves from prejudices because we are usually not aware that we are prejudiced; it requires a consistent effort to recognize when we are reacting to other people on the basis of preconceived ideas rather than in terms of each specific individual and situation. No one can live in this country today and not be aware of the existence and the tragic results of prejudice against all of our minority groups. It is our responsibility as decent human beings and as citizens of a democracy to do all that we can to end this cruel state of affairs—and the first place to start is with ourselves.

There is another way in which we can be prejudiced—it may not be tragic, but it is always unfair. We hear a comment at the lunch table that Miss A. or Mr. B. or Mrs. C. is a very poor worker. If one of these workers is later transferred to our service, we may not remember the exact comment, or who made it under what circumstances, but even before we observe this co-worker's performance, we think, "I know this worker isn't going to do good work. I don't know exactly why I think so, but I just know it." This is prejudice, too, and the worker is at a great disadvantage before he ever starts to work.

Stereotypes and prejudices may block our interpersonal relationships. There are many ways, however, in which a positive influence may be created by the nurse's behavior. Foremost among these, and too often overlooked, is the effect of treating clients and co-workers with courtesy. By behaving politely toward a person, regardless of his age, his cultural background, his education, or his economic status, we show at once that we respect him as an individual. It is easy, of course, to behave courteously when we in turn are treated with courtesy; it is more difficult when we are faced with hostility and rudeness. The important thing to remember is that our purpose is to establish an effective relationship and as teachers we must take the initiative toward this goal. Acting only on the basis of how other people treat us and keeping "company manners" just for certain people and certain situations will severely limit our relationships. Good manners on the part of the nurse will often smooth many otherwise difficult paths and will often produce similar behavior on the part of the learner, thus paving the way for developing good rapport.

The fostering of good relationships may also be favorably influenced if the nurse realizes that the teacher can learn from the learner, sometimes about things completely apart from concepts of health or illness. By learning from the patient or co-worker, the practitioner can profit from the learner's knowledge, common interests will contribute to the relationship, and the learner will feel that he is giving as well as receiving.

The effect of this feeling of giving is especially important with patients. During acute illness, the nurse-patient relationship is likely to be characterized by feelings of helplessness on the part of the patient; this feeling has certain therapeutic value when the patient must be entirely dependent on the nurse. However, when the patient begins to recover and must start to take responsibility for himself, when he is ready to learn how to take care of himself, this feeling of helplessness may be a barrier to learning. It is important that the dependent nurse-patient relationship be replaced by the cooperative teacher-learner relationship. The nurse who is able to accept and encourage the patient's need to give after so much receiving will help in this transition.

We have discussed here some of the principles of establishing a good nurse-learner relationship; whatever the practitioner does to facilitate good rapport is likely to contribute to the cooperative effort that is necessary for successful teaching and learning.

Principle 2. Teaching Requires Effective Communication

In effective communication, an idea is transmitted by one person and received and correctly interpreted by another. In verbal communication, whether spoken or written, the medium of exchange is language. If there is to be correct interpretation of the communication, the receiver must know what meaning the sender attaches to the words he uses. One of the most common problems of communication in everyday life is that we assume that other people use words in just the same way we do; we make no attempt to define our words because we are not aware of any need to do so.

If terms are not defined, the listener is sometimes forced to make a choice among several possible meanings; the choice he makes will depend upon his previous knowledge and experience. For example, suppose a friend tells you he is moving to Portland. If you live in or near the New England states, you may assume that he is moving to Portland, Maine; if you live on the west coast, to Portland, Oregon; you might also assume he is going to any one of a dozen other towns named Portland in the United States, or to a city in Canada, in England, or Australia. If your friend says, "I'm moving to Portland, Oregon," he has defined his term and his meaning is clear. There will be no misunderstanding because you will not have had to make any assumptions.

As practitioners teaching all kinds of people from all kinds of backgrounds, it is essential to know what meaning our learners attach to the words they use and how they interpret the words we use. Even "ordinary" words like *soon, almost, near* have different meanings to different people. It is not enough, for example, to instruct a patient to do a prescribed exercise "frequently." Perhaps to you that means three or four times a day; it may mean once a day or once an hour to the patient. There must be mutual understanding. Having the patient tell you in his own words how often he is to do the exercise will make his interpretation of the word clear. Words must be used carefully and should be defined when there is any possibility of misunderstanding.

The teaching-learning situation is also affected by nonverbal communication; this kind of communication is most often unconscious behavior. The facial expressions, gestures, and general physical behavior of the learner may provide cues to the nurse as to how well the patient is learning. These cues can be especially helpful if the learner is a person who does not or cannot express himself easily in words. At the same time, the teacher is giving the learner nonverbal cues: a shrug of the shoulder or a sigh, or a spontaneous smile and a nod, can tell the learner either that the nurse is bored with this whole business of teaching or, on the other hand, that the patient is making good progress at the moment. Problems resulting from nonverbal communications are common, partly because we are very often unaware of our nonverbal behavior and partly because this behavior is so obvious to anyone who looks at us.

In the following chapter on the learners, a section is devoted to problems in communication. In all situations, effective communication is essential for both teaching and learning; it is the responsibility of the practitioner to be sure that the two-way channel between teacher and learner is always open.

Principle 3. Learning Needs of Clients and Co-workers Must Be Determined

In many educational settings, the teacher knows in advance what the learners need to be taught. For example, in the primary grades, the teacher knows that most pupils need to learn to read and write, to spell, to count; in later grades, subject matter is definitely prescribed in history, science, or mathematics. This does not mean that adjustments do not have to be made for individual learners, but teachers in schools know in general what their prospective pupils have already learned. In teaching about health and illness, however, the nursing practitioner faces a different situation. Some clients will be quite sophisticated about health principles, others may have only the most rudimentary knowledge; some will have had extensive experience with illness, others may have had none. Before any plans for teaching can be made, the nurse must determine what the client's previous learning and experience has been and what he still needs to be taught. Teaching what the learner already knows is wasteful of time and energy for both the nurse and the client, and in addition can make the learner feel that his intelligence is being questioned. Teaching more than the learner needs to know or teaching things that are irrelevant can be very frustrating to him. In either case, we fail to meet his learning needs.

There are numerous ways to determine what the learner needs to know. First, the learner may be aware himself of gaps in his knowledge and may specifically ask for information. Second, by listening attentively, the nurse may discover some of these gaps by comments the learner makes or questions he asks. Third, the nurse may observe behavior which shows a need for learning. Fourth, the nurse may ask questions of the learner. These are all direct methods of determining learning needs.

There are indirect ways of securing this information, but they must be used with caution and good judgment, because they involve assumptions which should not be accepted as valid unless there is evidence to prove they are justified. Some examples may illustrate this point. Notice that in each case the word *may* is used in the assumption; the nurse should develop the habit of withholding judgment in making inferences about learning needs. Even when the inference is almost sure to be correct, decisions must be based on facts, not on assumptions.

A patient who has recently been discovered to have diabetes *may* need to be taught the relation of insulin to metabolism; he *may* need to be taught how to give himself insulin. The mother who brings an under-nourished child to the clinic *may* need to be taught basic information about nutrition; she *may* need to be taught how to shop for food more economically. The nursing aide who is observed doing a procedure incorrectly *may* need to be taught the entire technique again; he *may* need to be given an opportunity for further practice under supervision.

The main point to be learned from this discussion is that the practitioner must distinguish carefully between facts and assumptions. Assumptions and inferences are of great value in teaching when they are used as a guide for securing more information; they can be detrimental if they are treated as though they were facts.

Both direct and indirect methods may be used effectively in determining what the learner needs to be taught about health and illness. The practitioner must assess the client's learning needs before specific plans for teaching can be made.

Principle 4. Objectives Serve as Guides in Planning and Evaluating Teaching

When the learning needs of the client have been discovered, a plan for teaching him what he needs to know has to be developed. The first step in this plan is the formulation of objectives. An objective is the goal or purpose of an activity; in this case, it is a statement of what the practitioner hopes to accomplish in teaching this client.

Objectives are not limited to teaching; we are continually setting objectives for ourselves in our daily lives, even though we may not consciously label them as objectives. For example, a very specific, short-term objective we might set for ourselves is to get to a particular place at a definite time to keep an appointment; a broader objective might be to learn a skill, such as dancing or swimming; an inclusive, long-term objective might be to become a nurse. Thus, an objective is a goal we set for ourselves that implies a plan of action.

There are three important reasons for formulating objectives. The first is to make clear exactly what is to be accomplished. To fail to clarify our purpose is comparable to going to a bus terminal and asking the agent for a ticket without stating our destination. Of course, if our objective is just to get away from the place where we are, any ticket will do; on the other hand, if we have a specific goal in mind, we will have to buy a ticket to a particular destination. This is just as true for teaching; if we want to teach effectively, we must know exactly what our purpose is each time we plan to teach.

The second reason for clarifying objectives is that well-formulated goals serve as guides for planning action; they give direction. Consider the simple objective mentioned earlier of keeping an appointment. Suppose the purpose of the appointment is to have an interview for a job. How does this clarification help me to plan my actions? It will guide me in deciding how I will dress, what papers I will take with me, what time I should leave home to arrive in plenty of time, what route I must take to get to the right place. Now, suppose the purpose of the appointment is to meet some friends to go to the beach. The same questions will be raised, but the answers will be quite different. It is clear that the very general objective of keeping an appointment does not give much direction for planning, but when the objective is expanded to include the nature of the appointment, the course of action becomes much clearer.

The third reason for establishing objectives is that they serve as the key to the evaluation of teaching and learning. This purpose will be discussed in more detail when we consider evaluation in a later chapter.

To turn now to the practitioner's objectives in teaching, the nurse may state the objective of the teaching function as "to help people learn about health and illness." True, this is the overall goal of the practitioner's teaching, but, as it is stated, it is too general and vague to give any direction as to how this teaching is to be accomplished. To be of real value, objectives must be formulated for a particular area of teaching, a definite topic, and even for a specific learner. Let us assume that the nurse works in a prenatal clinic and see how the overall objective of helping people learn about health and illness might be clarified so that it will be of practical use in the nurse's planning for teaching. The following list of objectives shows how the general objective might be modified. It is important to note that in no case does an objective on the list contradict the overall objective and that in every case each objective is more limited and specific than the one that precedes it. The sequence begins with the overall objective, proceeds to a circumscribed area of teaching, then to a general topic, a specific lesson, and a particular learner. The material in parentheses indicates the progressive limitation of the objectives.

1. To help people learn about health and illness
   (A general objective for all nursing practitioners)
2. To help pregnant women learn about health and illness
   (A general objective for all practitioners working with pregnant women, whether in clinics, doctors' offices, or public health agencies)

3. To help prenatal patients learn about the need for regular physical examinations during pregnancy
   (A more specific objective for nurses working with prenatal patients)
4. To help patients attending this clinic to understand the significance of excessive weight gain and the importance of treatment
   (An even more specific objective for nurses working in a particular clinic)
5. To help Mrs. A, who is showing early symptoms of toxemia, to understand why it is important for her to attend the clinic regularly
   (A completely specific objective for a specific situation)

By means of this formulation of objectives, the nurse has proceeded in gradual steps from the general objective of the teaching function of all nursing practitioners to an objective that will meet a specific learning situation for Mrs. A. It is important to note that this objective is very limited and covers only as much as we might hope to teach Mrs. A in a brief conference. If Mrs. A has other learning needs, which will probably be the case, they may be covered by other objectives in other conferences.

How does this clarification of objectives help the nurse plan for teaching Mrs. A? First, it shows clearly what content will be covered: signs and symptoms of toxemia, need for early treatment, importance of regular physical examinations, and so forth. Second, the method of teaching is implied: an individual conference with the patient. Third, teaching materials appropriate to the objective suggest themselves: pamphlets on prenatal care, a schedule of prenatal clinic hours, and so on. The objective does not predict exactly how the teaching will be done, but it does suggest ideas for content, methods, and materials for the practitioner's consideration.

Objectives may be classified in various ways (central, concomitant, contributory) or may be divided into teacher's aims and students' aims. It is suggested that for the practitioner's teaching, they be classified solely as *teacher's objectives* and be stated in terms of the practitioner's goals for the learner. It is also suggested that the stated objectives begin with verbs (in the infinitive form) that suggest the nurse's helping function; for example, to help the patient to learn to care for himself; to enable the family member to carry out this procedure at home; to assist the nursing aide to understand the principles of asepsis.

In summary, objectives serve to give the practitioner direction in planning for teaching and evaluating learning. After the client's learning needs have been determined, the formulation of objectives is the first step in organizing teaching.

Principle 5. Planning Time for Teaching and Learning
Requires Special Attention

In the typical school situation, blocks of time are scheduled in advance by school administrators, the students and the teacher meet in an assigned classroom, and the alloted time is devoted to teaching and learning, the primary purpose of the school; there is seldom interruption because of other responsibilities of the teacher or the students. This is not the case in most nursing situations for several reasons.

First, the primary purpose of nursing services is the care of the sick and this function takes precedence over all others. It is true that frequently emphasis is placed on the teaching function of public health and school nurses, but even here when the occasion demands it, the care of the sick has priority over teaching. It is reasonable, therefore, that specific teaching time is not scheduled by most nursing service administrators, particularly in hospitals and outpatient departments, and it becomes the responsibility of the practitioner to plan such time.

Second, as we pointed out previously, teaching is only one aspect of the nurse's responsibilities. In the ongoing activities of a busy nursing service, the nurse may have many duties to perform for a large number of patients and be subject to frequent interruptions. The problems of planning time for teaching in such situations are apparent.

Third, there are numerous interruptions and distractions for the learners. In the hospital setting, because of the patient's need for diagnostic tests and special therapies, he may spend a good deal of time away from the nursing unit in other areas of the hospital and thus not be available when the nurse has time to teach. Increasingly short hospital stays also add to the problem of arranging time for patient teaching. Planning time for teaching auxiliary personnel either in the hospital or in the public health agency is complicated by the fact that these workers have a responsibility for ongoing patient care which necessarily occupies most of their time. Nurses who work in clinics and doctors' offices, in homes and schools, have a different problem: clients in these settings do not constitute a captive audience as do patients in the hospital; they are involved in their own personal lives and interests and may be unable or unwilling to plan with the nurse for time for learning what they need to know about their health.

In spite of these difficulties, the resourceful nurse can often devise ways of planning time for teaching. First, although we have said that arranging time for teaching in advance may often be very difficult, it should not be assumed to be impossible. Close attention to the patient's activities for the day or the auxiliary worker's assignment may make it possible to find time mutually convenient for both nurse and learner. When time is available it should be used to the best possible advantage.

The learner should know what is going to be discussed and when possible be given pamphlets or other printed materials on the topic so that he will be ready; the nurse should be well prepared and have teaching materials on hand so that time will not be wasted.

A great deal of teaching can be done while the practitioner is carrying out other nursing functions. A patient can be taught as the nurse is giving him physical care; a nursing assistant can be taught while the nurse is supervising his work. On some occasions the nurse may be able to teach several clients at once; for example, a group of patients with similar learning needs who attend a clinic at the same time may be taught in a group.

Time affects the nurse's plans for teaching in another way. It requires time to teach and time to learn, but even a very experienced teacher cannot predict exactly how much time will be necessary in a particular situation. The nurse must try to be flexible in planning the time element and not expect that a certain topic can be presented in exactly thirty minutes or that a learner can master a given amount of subject matter in a specified time. The nurse will also discover that several short periods of teaching are sometimes more effective than one long period, just as several short, spaced practice periods for the learner are more likely to be productive than one long session.

Factors in nursing settings create many problems in relation to the time element in teaching, but a certain amount of ingenuity and the careful planning and use of available time will help in some measure to solve the problem which must be overcome in order for teaching to be accomplished.

Principle 6. Control of the Environment Is an Aspect of Teaching

Factors in the physical environment where teaching is to be done can contribute to a pleasant and effective learning situation or can make learning extremely difficult or impossible. Adequate ventilation and temperature, good lighting, and appropriate furniture will contribute to the physical comfort of the learner and the teacher, and, incidentally, may set an example of good health practices. Freedom from noise and other distractions is important; if possible, a separate room closed off from the activities of the ward, the clinic, or the home should be used. When this cannot be done, teaching should be scheduled at times when there is a minimum of interference. Necessary equipment should be available and easily accessible and there must be adequate space in which to use it. In the patient's home, where standard equipment is often not at hand, plans must be made for improvising from materials that are available. It is sometimes impossible to control some of the factors in the physical environment, but the practitioner should try to do all that can be done to make the setting conducive to learning.

Principle 7. Learning Principles Must Be Applied Appropriately

In the discussion of the principles of learning in the last chapter, examples were given of the application of principles to nursing situations. In order to apply these principles appropriately, the nurse must consider the particular learner in the specific situation and attempt to evaluate as accurately as possible exactly what he brings to this learning situation, to assess his assets and liabilities as far as learning is concerned, and to plan how best to help him learn effectively. As we become acquainted with this learner and establish rapport with him, we will be able to answer some of the questions that will give us help in adapting our teaching to his needs.

For example, here are some questions we might ask ourselves. Is the learner's physical and emotional condition such that he can concentrate on learning now? Does he have difficulties in perception that may interfere with learning? Is he motivated to learn? Does he have good health habits which should be reinforced? Is he physically and mentally capable of learning? If not, should someone in his family be taught about his care? Do we know enough about his previous knowledge and experience to teach on a level that will be challenging to him? Are we prepared to accept his mistakes as part of the process of learning and to be patient in answering his questions? Have we planned to allow enough time for practice and for as much repetition as he needs? Do our own health habits set an example we want him to imitate? How shall we involve him actively in learning?

In applying the principles of learning appropriately, the nurse must of necessity know the general principles as they relate to all learning, but in the final analysis, successful teaching depends on the practitioner's ability to plan and carry out teaching in accordance with the needs of each unique, individual learner.

Principle 8. Teaching Skill Can Be Acquired Through Practice and Observation

The teaching techniques appropriate in nursing settings will be discussed in detail in a later chapter, but at this point we can make some general comments about developing teaching skill. The nurse who is learning to teach is involved in the same process as the client who is learning about health and illness; the same principles of learning are operating. Consider these principles from the viewpoint of the prospective teacher of health in the role of a learner.

The nurse must be motivated toward teaching; a genuine interest in helping people learn and an acceptance of the importance of the practitioner's teaching function will provide that motivation. The development of teaching skill requires that the nurse become actively involved in trying to teach, in getting frequent practice, and in repeating the practice many times to improve teaching skill. Just as the nurse expects the client or co-worker to use trial-and-error learning at times and to make mistakes, errors will be made in learning to teach; but if a conscientious attempt is made to determine what errors were made and why they were made, the nurse can profit from mistakes.

During the process of learning to teach, the nurse will find it helpful to observe more experienced practitioners as they teach and to discuss with them the problems of teaching that inevitably arise even in skillful teaching. Another way to learn by observation is by means of television, either by watching expert teachers on educational television channels or by observing techniques used by interviewers or public speakers on commercial channels. It is important to remember that it can be useful to observe poor techniques as well as good ones, providing that the nurse analyzes why some techniques were not effective in the situations in which they were used.

Interest in teaching, willingness to try to teach, analysis of one's own and other people's performance, and the ability to ask for and accept suggestions will all contribute to the development of teaching skill.

Principle 9. Evaluation Is an Integral Part of Teaching

Evaluation is the appraisal of the outcomes of an activity. In teaching, it is the process by which the teacher attempts to arrive at an objective judgment of the effectiveness of teaching. It involves an analysis of both teaching and learning and is a systematic and ongoing process. Without sound evaluation, the practitioner has no way of knowing with certainty that the teaching is producing the desired learning. This principle will be discussed in detail in the chapter on evaluating teaching and learning.

SUMMARY

The principles of teaching presented in this chapter are restated here as a summary.
1. Good nurse-learner rapport is important in teaching.
2. Teaching requires effective communication.
3. Learning needs of clients and co-workers must be determined.
4. Objectives serve as guides in planning and evaluating teaching.
5. Planning time for teaching and learning requires special attention.
6. Control of the environment is an aspect of teaching.

7. Learning principles must be applied appropriately.
8. Teaching skill can be acquired through practice and observation.
9. Evaluation is an integral part of teaching.

The references on the principles of learning suggested at the end of the previous chapter contain valuable material about principles of teaching, since learning and teaching are so closely related. The student might benefit from reviewing some of those references from the point of view of the teacher, in addition to the references listed below.

REFERENCES

AICHLMAYR, RITA HOESCHEN. "Cultural Understanding: A Key to Acceptance." *Nursing Outlook* 17:20-23, July, 1969.
The author points out the error of equating minority status or low economic status with cultural deprivation and describes experiences of public health nursing students working with Indians on a reservation in northern Washington state. With understanding of their patients' cultures and values, the nurses could give more meaningful service.

BACA, JOSEPHINE ELIZABETH. "Some Health Beliefs of the Spanish Speaking." *American Journal of Nursing* 69:2172-76, October, 1969.
This article has value for all nurses, whether or not they work with the people the author writes about, to remind us that all of us probably have some "folk medicine" beliefs, regardless of our origins.

HALL, EDWARD T. *The Silent Language.* Greenwich, Conn.: Fawcett Publications, 1963.
This book touching on the lack of understanding among people of different cultures has many implications for the nurse in teaching people of various cultural backgrounds.

HAYAKAWA, S. I. *Language in Thought and Action*, 2d ed. New York: Harcourt, Brace & World, Inc., 1964.
This book is a classic in the field of semantics—the study of the meaning and use of words. It is a thought-provoking and entertaining book that the reader will find useful in personal as well as professional life.

LEVINE, DALE C., and FIEDLER, JUNE P. "Fears, Facts and Fantasies About Pre- and Postoperative Care." *Nursing Outlook* 18:26-28, February, 1970.
The authors describe teaching patients and their families about what to expect pre- and postoperatively. They have found that teaching has helped the patients, the families, and the nurses while the patient is in the recovery room or intensive care unit.

LEWIS, GARLAND K. *Nurse-Patient Communication.* 2d ed. Dubuque, Iowa: Wm. C. Brown Company Publishers, 1973.
The reader will find in this book a thorough discussion of communications between nurse and patient, which can be applied also to the teacher-learner relationship.

TRAVELBEE, JOYCE. "What's Wrong with Sympathy?" *American Journal of Nursing* 64:68-71, January, 1964.
The author expresses the idea that without compassion and sympathy, the nurse limits herself to "interaction" with patients and cannot develop a truly supportive relationship.

WOODRUFF, ASAHEL D. *Basic Concepts of Teaching,* concise ed. San Francisco: Chandler Publishing Company, 1962.
  The reader's attention is called to the list of educational concepts in the introduction to this book and to the chapters on the teaching of concepts and motor skills and changing habits.

Chapter _____ 4

The Learners

In this chapter we will discuss the most important people involved in the practitioner's teaching—the learners. Without them, there would be no need to teach; with them, whether we succeed or fail in our teaching depends on whether or not they learn. All potential learners (that is, *all* human beings) are complex individuals; when the learners are also patients, or their families, or the workers who take care of them, there are additional complexities. If the nurse is able to develop a good understanding of these learners and how their lives are affected by illness or by close association with those who are ill, teaching and learning may be more effective.

We will summarize briefly some factors in the nursing setting that may affect the learner, or the teacher, or both, and thus influence the outcome of our teaching efforts; then we will look at the learners and see how they may differ from learners in other situations.

FACTORS IN NURSING SETTINGS THAT AFFECT TEACHING AND LEARNING

The chief factor that influences the practitioner's teaching is the nature of the learner: his physical and emotional state; his age, his social and cultural background, his education and experience; the voluntary nature of the client's relationship to the nurse as a teacher.

The second factor is the nature of nursing itself: the fact that nursing care has priority over teaching; the great variety of nursing settings, some of which do not lend themselves easily to teaching; the problem of planning time for teaching along with all the other nursing activities that must be scheduled.

The third factor is the nature of the practitioner's functions: the nurse's role in providing patient care and supervising nursing assistants; the responsibility to the physician for carrying out medical orders; the many other duties that are part of the nurse's functions.

In the following sections of this chapter, the discussion of the specific problems of teaching and learning in nursing settings will be organized in terms of the nature of the learners. Concerns relating to the nature of nursing and the nature of the practitioner's functions will be included where they have relevance.

Emphasis has been placed in the preceding chapters on the uniqueness of each learner and the need to recognize individual differences. In this chapter we will be looking at *common* problems of groups of learners. Common problems exist because the people involved are subject to common physical, emotional, experiential, or environmental factors that tend to produce similar effects. It is important to recall here the dangers of generalizing and stereotyping: problems that are common to a group of people do not necessarily occur in every member of the group. Thus our discussion will point up problems that particular groups may have or are likely to have; the nurse must always try to determine whether or not these problems do, in fact, exist for the particular learner in a specific situation. The learners will be classified as follows: (1) patients in various stages of illness, (2) patients who have problems in communicating, (3) clients in good health, (4) nursing co-workers supervised by the practitioner, and (5) co-workers in schools and industry.

PATIENTS IN VARIOUS STAGES OF ILLNESS

The learners to be discussed here are patients who are acutely ill, patients with long-term illness, convalescent patients, and patients in the clinic or doctor's office and in the home.

Patients Who Are Acutely Ill

During acute illness it is unlikely that any teaching or learning can be accomplished. At this time the patient's goal is physical survival and all his body's resources are focused in this direction. Pain, mental confusion, debilitation, fear, anxiety are all factors which may accompany acute illness and preclude any attempts at teaching. Even when the patient is temporarily free of these symptoms, the need for rest and sleep is paramount. This is clearly one of the times when the function of giving nursing care must take precedence over teaching.

Patients with Long-Term Illness

Several factors may be operating in long-term illness that will have an effect on teaching and learning. Of primary importance is the patient's reaction to the reality of his illness. The prospect of prolonged or permanent physical incapacity can have a devastating effect on the individual. In addition to the physical aspects of the illness, the patient faces a threat to his image of himself as a functioning, independent person, the impact of a changed way of life on himself and perhaps on his family, and the financial problems that are usually involved. Some patients may be able to work out these conflicts by their own efforts; others may express their frustration by open aggression, by withdrawal, or by apparent indifference.

The aggressive patient is likely to take out his feelings on the nurse. It is very difficult in any situation not to react negatively to hostility, excessive demands and complaints, or unending appeals for attention and sympathy, but it is important to realize that such behavior may be symptomatic of the patient's inner conflict. The patient's expression of his frustration may be the first step in resolving the conflicts. The nurse who can accept these reactions calmly and pay attention to what the patient is saying (and what he avoids saying) may be able to discover a good deal about his underlying problems and use this information constructively for his benefit.

The withdrawn or apparently indifferent patient is difficult to help because he retreats into silence and may be unable to ask for help or to accept it when it is offered. Moreover, since he is so quiet, he may be overlooked on a busy nursing unit where more aggressive patients are demanding the nurse's attention. If the practitioner's attempts to establish contact with these patients are unsuccessful, the doctor should be notified; more expert help than the nurse has been prepared to give may be needed.

Just as the acutely ill person cannot concentrate on learning because of his physical problems, the patient who is trying to resolve his conflicts about accepting long-term illness cannot concentrate on learning until his emotional problems are under control.

Patients who have been chronically ill for a long time may present a problem to the teacher because they have been living with their illness for years and feel, justifiably or not, that they know more about it than anyone else. This is a situation in which the teacher might well become the learner, not only because the patient may indeed have something of value to teach the nurse about how he has learned to live with his illness, but because it is important for the patient to feel that he is able to contribute something to a relationship in which he is usually the receiver.

The very young patient and the elderly patient who have long-term illnesses present special problems simply because of their ages. The very young child will probably not be disturbed about the effect of his illness on his future life; it is the present that is most important to him. His major concern will probably be the restrictions his illness places on the normal activities of childhood, his inability to do the things his friends do. With some thought and a little ingenuity, the nurse can provide him with quiet but interesting and absorbing things to do to occupy him during the period when he is adjusting to the necessary changes in his pattern of living. When the child has been able to accept the reality of his illness to some extent, it will be time enough to begin to teach him the principles of hygiene and health related to his illness.

At the other end of the age range are the geriatric patients, who constitute the largest proportion of people with long-term illness and whose number is steadily increasing because of the medical advances which prolong life. Patients in their advancing years have emotional needs, of course, but their ability to satisfy these needs may be severely limited because of their age and their illness. They can no longer be independent as they once were, they may have doubts about being wanted and needed by their families and friends, their former ability to achieve and to receive recognition may have diminished; all these changes in their life patterns are likely to lead to a serious loss of self-respect and a feeling of hopelessness. Added to this is the realization, openly expressed or deeply hidden, that life is nearly over for them. It is no wonder that these patients are often overwhelmed by their problems and may manifest their hurt and frustration in aggressive or withdrawing behavior.

Helping the older patient to regain his feeling of worth and self-esteem is not easy and cannot be accomplished quickly. It requires a real understanding and acceptance of the patient's "difficult" behavior, the development of a relationship in which the patient knows that the nurse is sincerely interested in him as a person, and consistent efforts by the nurse to encourage and give recognition to any attempt by the patient to take responsibility for himself. For most of these patients it is probably best to teach on an informal, individual basis and to concentrate on teaching simple techniques of self-help.

The Convalescent Patient

As a rule, convalescent hospital patients are well motivated to learn because they want to return to their homes and resume their normal lives. Lack of interest in learning at this point may indicate reluctance to leave the hospital for any number of reasons and should probably be investigated further.

The teaching of the convalescent patient is, unfortunately, often neglected. It is unfortunate because this is the time when teaching and learning may be most effective. It is impossible to teach while the patient's life is in jeopardy, or while he is still very ill. It is during convalescence, when he and his family know that he is safe and everyone's emotions are under control, that the atmosphere lends itself to teaching and learning. It is important that the teaching be started as soon as it is feasible, since in these days of short hospital stays patients go home for most of their convalescence.

There are several logical reasons, but few valid excuses, for the frequent failure to teach the convalescent patient: the crisis is over, recovery has begun, the patient can bathe and dress and feed himself, the family will soon be taking him home. Sometimes when we have a convalescent on our patient assignment, we go in and say, "Good morning," continue with some small talk while we make the bed and straighten the unit, and mentally check him off as we proceed to other patients "who *really* need nursing care." If the phrase in quotation marks did not bother you when you read it, it would be wise for you to do some thinking about it. You are equating *physical care* with *nursing care*. Sometimes we have to remind ourselves, particularly on a very busy service where we have a lot to do, that the patient is more than just the physical being in the bed, especially when the medical crisis is over.

Why is this convalescent period so important for the patient? Suppose we take a "patient's-eye view" of his recent experiences. Let us assume that our patient is a businessman in his late fifties who "never had a sick day in his life." He has had a heart attack at work and has been rushed to the hospital by ambulance. In the space of an hour, he has experienced the terror of the heart attack, the confusion of the ambulance ride, and then the sudden and utter dependence upon doctors and nurses, and those machines in the cardiac intensive care unit. When the major crisis is over, he is transferred to the ward, where he is still dependent on someone else for his intimate bodily care—a grown man who has been active in the business world, supporting a family, sending his children to college. It is no wonder that he may have difficulty in adjusting to the dependent role—he has to learn to be a patient. And after he accomplishes this, what may happen? The doctor may say that he is well enough to get out of bed for part of the day and begin to take care of himself; now he has to "un-learn" being a patient. After perhaps several weeks of total dependence in order to survive, he is suddenly expected to be self-sufficient, in spite of the terrifying memory of that heart attack hanging over his head like a cloud. He has been the focus of attention of his family and friends and the hospital staff—and suddenly this is no longer true. It makes no difference that he is a grown man—he feels the change and it may hurt, frighten, bewilder, or anger him, or produce a combination of feelings. Added to that, he may not recognize these feelings or, if he does, he tries to ignore or suppress them because "no grown man should feel this way." The usual warning is in order for the nurse: *we must not assume* the patient is feeling any particular way; we must try to find out how he has responded, and help him express these feelings. This is the nursing care this patient needs, and he needs it just as much as the patient down the hall needs physical care. It is important to remember that, although we have had experience caring for ten or a hundred or five hundred patients recovering from heart attacks, this is the *first* experience for this patient. Helping him accept the need to resume his independence is essential if he is to be able to learn other things we want to teach him during his convalescence.

The Patient in the Clinic or the Doctor's Office

Opportunities and facilities for teaching are similar in clinics and doctors' offices. In general, planning in advance is possible since the nurse usually knows beforehand which patients are scheduled for appointments, medical charts are at hand, and the doctor can be easily contacted if there is a question about what the patient should be taught. Sometimes in a particular clinic or the office of a doctor who is a specialist, group teaching may be appropriate for patients who have similar learning needs. Since the nurse is likely to be very busy during the time when the doctor is seeing patients, it may be necessary to arrange for teaching before clinic or office hours while the patients are waiting to see the doctor or after appointments have been completed. At the same time the practitioner must be realistic about the amount of time the patients will be able or willing to spend for this purpose.

Since the practitioner's contact with these patients is intermittent, in contrast to the daily contact with patients in the hospital, special efforts must be made to insure continuity by careful planning and reviewing with the patient what has already been taught.

The Patient in the Home

The problems of acute and chronic illness and convalescence which we have just discussed have the same impact on the patient in the home as on the patient in the hospital, but there are other factors in the home setting that may affect teaching and learning.

Perhaps the chief difference in teaching in the home is that here the nurse is a visitor. In the hospital we expect the patient and his family to conform to hospital rules; in the home it is the nurse who makes the adjustments. The disruption of household activities is not conducive to maintaining good relationships. It takes very little effort to arrange with the family for the best time to visit and this planning may make the difference between accomplishing the purpose of the visit or being resisted as an unwelcome intruder.

There are other aspects of teaching in the home which may be planned with the patient or his family. If there is a choice of rooms that might be used, the family should be consulted as to which room would be most convenient in relation to the regular household activities, adequate space for the teaching that is to be done, and convenience to kitchen or bathroom facilities. If the plans for teaching include a procedure that requires special equipment that the family is expected to provide, or the adaptation of household articles, this should be discussed in advance if possible, so that the family will not be made uncomfortable because things are not on hand and the nurse will not have to inconvenience the family or devote the limited time available to assembling materials that are needed.

Successful teaching in the home is based in large measure on establishing good relationships with the members of the household and securing the cooperation of the family as well as the patient in planning for teaching.

PATIENTS WHO HAVE PROBLEMS IN COMMUNICATING

Learning will be difficult if not impossible when there are serious blocks in communication between teacher and learner. As in any problem-solving situation, the practitioner must first realize that there is a problem, identify and define it, and then attempt to reach a solution. It is important to understand the significance of the phrase, "realize that there is a problem." In many instances problems in communicating with patients are not immediately apparent. For example, patients who do not realize that they are becoming deaf actually may not know that they are not hearing correctly what is said to them; a patient who does not speak English but who has discovered that the word "yes" will generally bring a positive response, may say "yes" whenever the nurse's tone of voice indicates that an answer is expected, even though he may have no idea of what has been said. On the other side is the nurse who mumbles; the nurse who uses difficult words or technical words and assumes that the patient understands; the nurse who turns what should be a simple teaching incident into a lecture, doing all the talking and sometimes frightening or boring the patient into silence when he should be taking an active part. If the nurse fails to recognize that something is wrong in the communication, it is probable that any learning that takes place will be in spite of, not because of, the nurse.

The practitioner must be alert to recognize signs of misunderstanding or confusion: facial expressions, questions by the patient that show that he does not understand what has been said, lack of attention. Very often in nursing situations, when inadequate communication has been identified and the cause determined, there is no simple solution. Deafness, blindness, inability to speak English, inability to speak at all—the practitioner cannot correct these problems, of course, but it is sometimes possible to circumvent them so that our patients can learn what it is important for them to know. We will discuss some of these problems with two purposes in mind: first, the better understanding of how these communications problems affect the patient and, second, some of the ways in which we can cross the communication barrier.

The Patient Who Cannot Hear and the Patient Who Cannot Speak

Patients who cannot hear and those who cannot speak are included together here because there is a certain similarity between the problems these two groups have in communicating. We have spoken earlier of what is required for communication: a sender, a mode of transmission, and a receiver. In the case of the deaf person, the sender (the nurse) is there, a mode of transmission (the voice) is there, but the patient cannot receive the message. In the case of those who cannot speak, the sender (the patient) is there, but the mode of transmission is missing so that the nurse cannot receive the message. It is true that the person who has lost his hearing may learn to read lips at some future time and the person who no longer has a larynx may eventually learn esophageal speech. However, the nurse often works with these patients before they have had time to learn these new skills and often while they are still experiencing the psychological shock that accompanies the permanent loss of hearing or of normal speech.

The nurse should try earnestly to get at least some insight into the frustrations of such handicaps. You may appreciate these problems better by trying two simple experiments. First, the next time you want particularly to watch a certain television program, tune in the set and turn off the sound. See how long you can endure the frustration before you end the experiment by turning up the sound. (Be sure to choose a program you really *want* to view.) Second, spend a social evening with some friends and do not speak a word, even to explain the experiment. Again, see how long you can stand it. (Be sure that neither you nor your friends make a game out of it.) After these experiences, think about the fact that when the frustrations become just about unbearable, the deaf person cannot turn up the sound and the person who is not able to speak cannot easily make explanations—*their* physical problems are permanent.

These experiments may give you further understanding of these difficulties if you will recall what bothered you particularly. Was it having someone turn away from the television camera so that you could not even tell whether they were speaking, let alone receive any cues as to what they were saying from seeing their mouths move or watching their facial expressions? If you used paper and pencil when you were not allowing yourself to speak, was there added irritation because you ran out of paper, or broke the pencil point, or because someone wrote his answers, thinking for the moment that since you were not speaking, you could not hear? Whatever annoyances added to your frustration, remember them when you work with patients who have these problems, and act accordingly. If you are going to be successful in teaching these patients, it is you who must take the first and sometimes the larger step in establishing communication with them.

Although having to write down what you want to say is a slow and tiresome procedure, it may be the best solution when the nurse is working with patients who cannot hear or patients who cannot speak. A "magic slate" or small notebook and pencil tied to the frame of the bed with long strings will be very useful. The strings are important since they make it easy to retrieve slates or pads or pencils that fall on the floor or get lost in the bed clothes.

There are several points that the nurse should keep in mind about *partially* deaf patients. In most instances, deafness is a condition that approaches very gradually. Many people who are becoming hard of hearing do not realize what is happening; this period can be very difficult for the individual as well as for those around him. Not being able to hear clearly is very frustrating for the patient, and having to repeat loudly every word that is said is very frustrating for everyone else. In order to establish and maintain good communication, the nurse must be quick to recognize the signs of partial deafness—the head turned and the hand cupped behind the "good" ear, the puzzled and sometimes angry expression on the face, the continual repetition, "What did you say?"

There is one more concept the nurse should be aware of about people who are deaf. It may seem to the person who can hear that deafness is an unfortunate but minor handicap. This is not true. Deaf people may often be in physical danger because they cannot hear car horns, fire alarms, police sirens, or even a warning, "Look out!" In addition to physical jeopardy, deafness may come to be a very serious handicap in terms of the patient's mental health. Because of the never-ending silence and the resulting social isolation, deaf people have been known to develop strong feelings of persecution, sometimes leading to paranoid psychosis. Lest you think that this is a far-fetched idea, try to recall the last time you were in a room with several people who were talking together in such low tones that you could not hear what they were saying. If they happened to glance in your direction, did it cross your mind, if only for an instant, that they were talking about *you*, and were talking softly because they were saying uncomplimentary things about you? If this happened to you day after day, would it be surprising if you began to develop the feeling that everyone was against you? Be sure, then, when you talk in the presence of a deaf patient, that he knows what the conversation is about. If you are talking with someone about something that is not the patient's concern, you should move out of the patient's field of vision.

The Patient Who Is Blind

The handicap of blindness interferes with communication in a very important but subtle way. Although the blind person can hear and speak, he is cut off from one of the fundamental avenues of social exchange—nonverbal communication. He can hear the words that are spoken, of course, but he cannot get the added messages, often more significant than the spoken words, that are conveyed by facial expressions, gestures, and body posture. We suggested earlier an experiment in which you viewed television with the sound turned off. Now turn up the sound and sit with your back to the set. You may begin to understand how much you depend on your eyes to tell you what a person *really* means by what he is saying. In this same connection, it is interesting that radio scripts and television scripts for dramatic programs cannot be interchanged, but must be rewritten, depending on whether the audience will only hear or will hear and also see the program.

Since we are primarily concerned here with teaching, we will mention some of the points to bear in mind when working with blind people; if our contacts are as comfortable as possible and show an understanding of at least some of the patient's problems, we will have established a good relationship for teaching and learning.

When you enter the room of a blind patient, make some sort of quiet sound so he will not be taken unaware, and introduce yourself by name at once. The patient will not be amused at being startled by your arrival or by being forced to play guessing games to identify you. Use your normal tone of voice (unless, of course, the patient also has a hearing loss); many people seem to try to cross the barrier of blindness by talking very loudly. If the patient is going to be out of bed, orient him to the room and its furniture and alert everyone who will be working in that room to replace furniture exactly, if they have to move it, lest the patient stumble or fall on furniture that is not where he was told it would be. Another hazard to the blind person is a half-open door; the patient may walk directly into the edge of it and injure his face; remind staff members to completely close or completely open all doors in the room. Be sure that whoever serves the patient his first tray asks him if he needs any help, and after giving this assistance, that the co-worker note on the chart or the Kardex what help the patient needs at mealtime.

Try to be aware of any sounds that may be strange to the patient and make it a habit to explain them. In the event of a ward emergency, be sure someone goes immediately to stay with the patient, even if he is not in actual danger, just so he knows what is happening and knows he has not been forgotten in case there *is* danger. Remember at all times to tell the patient you are leaving the room before doing so.

We have been discussing patients with certain physical handicaps. We have by no means included all such patients—that would be too extensive for this book. However, there is a very important point that must be raised about people with such handicaps before we leave this discussion. Most physically handicapped people who have lived with a handicap for a long time have become more or less adjusted to it. They do not want to be pitied and they do not appreciate being treated as though they were dependent children or "special cases." They have struggled to accept and live with their problem; they want you to accept it, too, and make only the adjustments required by their limitations. Aside from that, they want to be treated just as you would treat anyone else.

Attempts to communicate with patients who are deaf or hard of hearing or blind will sometimes be difficult and time-consuming for the nurse, but it is very important that you do not communicate impatience or annoyance even if you have these feelings—remember, it is the *patient* who has the big problem to live with, and he has more than enough to contend with already.

The Patient Who Does Not Speak English

The learner who does not speak English presents special problems. If the nurse can speak the learner's native tongue, the communication problem will, of course, be minimized; in addition, there will usually be very good rapport between teacher and learner, simply because the patient can understand and be understood. The phrase, "he speaks my language," is often used figuratively to express mutual understanding; in its literal sense, to speak someone else's language increases greatly the chances of such understanding.

In the absence of a mutual language, the help of an interpreter can be of great value, but if the interpreter is not a professional or a co-worker known to the nurse, the problem of communication is not automatically solved. The interpreter may be a family member or another patient whose own command of English is not very good. The nurse must be sure that the interpreter understands the nurse and that the patient understands the interpreter. Remember that very well-meaning people who want to help often volunteer to do a job, such as acting as interpreter, that they are not adequately prepared to do.

Without either a command of the learner's language or a dependable interpreter, a good deal of meaning can nevertheless be conveyed by the international language of gestures, facial expressions, and demonstrations. It is up to the nurse to exercise patience and ingenuity in establishing some kind of communication, even if all that is possible at first is to convey to the patient a feeling of acceptance and reassurance.

Two errors are often made in contacts with non-English-speaking people, neither of which is excusable for the practitioner. One error is to assume that because the learner cannot speak English he has a limited mentality. There is not necessarily any relationship between intelligence and the ability to speak English. The second error is to assume that the language barrier can be bridged by talking loudly. If the person does not understand the language, talking loudly will not help his comprehension and probably will add greatly to the frustration he already feels in not being able to understand or be understood. If we could imagine ourselves in a foreign country, sick, and in a hospital where no one speaks English, and then imagine ourselves being treated as if we were not very bright and being shouted at in a language we could not understand, we might have some idea of how a foreign-born person in this country would feel in similar circumstances.

There are several very simple but effective tools that can be used when no interpreter is available. Listed in a booklet or on cards, in English and in various other languages, are some of the usual questions and answers that nurses and patients would be likely to want to use. The phrase in English and in the various other languages has the same number, so that if the nurse wants to ask question 4, it is very easy to ask the patient by pointing to question 4 written in his language. The answers are given and translated in the same way. The Eli Lilly drug company publishes a free booklet *A Language Guide for Patient and Nurse* that contains translations of ten languages frequently encountered in the United States. The British Red Cross has designed a set of cards called *Language Cards for Hospital Patients* that includes thirty-two languages. These cards are available at a reasonable cost through the Office of International Relations of the American National Red Cross in Washington, D. C. Similar devices are available from other sources. Remember, too, that the nurse can make a set of such cards that apply to the particular situation the teacher and learner are in and have them translated into the languages most frequently encountered.

It really makes no difference what the source of the communication problem is—whether it is loss of hearing or sight or the inability to speak —in *any* situation, it is up to the practitioner to make every possible effort to establish two-way contact. If the approach is not, "Oh, he'll never understand!" but rather, "I'm sure I can get through if I just try hard enough," the practitioner will find that establishing communication in difficult situations will be a most rewarding experience.

CLIENTS IN GOOD HEALTH

The clients to be discussed here are the family of the hospitalized patient, the family in the home, children in schools, and employees in industry, expectant parents, parents of school children, and nursing students.

The Family of the Hospitalized Patient

The family of the patient who is acutely ill in the hospital will probably be no more amenable to teaching than the patient himself until his illness has subsided and he is on the road to recovery. Nevertheless, the nurse can become acquainted with the family when they visit the hospital and establish a relationship with them by trying to give them emotional support, by answering their questions, and by showing sincere interest in their concern for the patient. In this way, the nurse may gain some insight into the patient as a member of the family and also establish a good teacher-learner relationship with some member of the family who may have to help with the care of the patient on his release from the hospital. It is important that teaching the family about the patient's care begin as early as possible.

Opportunities for contact with the patient's family in the hospital may be limited. The nurse may have to plan for a specific time to see family members and arrange other nursing duties accordingly. If such arrangements are impractical, it may be necessary for the teaching to be done by the public health nurse who visits the home after the patient's discharge from the hospital. If a referral form is to be sent to the public health nursing agency, there should be a notation included to the effect that it was not possible to teach the family about the patient's care.

The Family in the Home

The alert nurse may find a number of opportunities for teaching in the home in relation to health problems of other members of the family or health or safety hazards in the home environment. It is one thing, however, to recognize such opportunities, but it is another matter to use them wisely. The saying about making haste slowly is most appropriate here. If the family members have been prepared for the nurse to come in to see the patient, they will usually welcome the visits. As a good relationship is gradually established with them and their confidence in the nurse develops, it may be possible to extend teaching to other areas. Perhaps the patient or someone in the family will ask a question or make a remark that will open the way, or the nurse may eventually broach the subject. The important thing is that the nurse must be very tactful in making suggestions about anything that is outside the original purpose of the visits, that is, caring for and teaching the patient. Suggestions should not imply negative criticism or unfavorable judgments by the practitioner; the family is likely to reject such suggestions and block the way for any further teaching.

Children in Schools and Employees in Industry

The practitioner's opportunities for teaching school children and industrial employees are similar, since in both instances the health program is centered in the medical or health office. Although the physician has the ultimate authority in the health office, it is the nurse who has the responsibility for the day-to-day routines and the opportunity to initiate plans for health supervision and teaching for pupils or employees.

The usual activities and procedures of the office provide an avenue for the nurse to get a general picture of the health problems and learning needs of individuals or of various groups. For example, medical records are available for pupils or employees, regular physical examinations are usually required, illness or injuries are reported, and clients who have been absent because of illness come to the health office before returning to classes or to work. Another very important source of information is the classroom teacher or the shop supervisor who has close contact with pupils or employees and may have suggestions for the health program. By pooling all this information, the nurse will be able to plan for meeting individual or group health needs. For example, a review of attendance or accident records may suggest the need for a campaign against colds for the third-graders or more emphasis on accident prevention for the men in the machine shop; a survey of the results of vision or hearing tests may indicate that these areas need attention, and so forth.

In addition to teaching individual pupils or employees when they visit the health office, it may be possible to schedule classes for groups of learners. In the school, the nurse may be responsible for teaching health education as part of the school curriculum or may act in an advisory capacity to classroom teachers who have this responsibility. In industry, it may be possible to arrange classes to teach such topics as first aid or plant safety. Whether or not health programs in schools and industry are effective depends to a large extent on the initiative and interest of the nurse in the health office.

Expectant Parents

The immediate objective in the teaching of expectant mothers and fathers is to promote the well-being of the mother and baby during pregnancy, delivery, and the postpartum period. The ultimate objective is to prepare these new parents for their responsibility for the health of their future family. Healthy parents and healthy infants are a good beginning for a family; parents who know how to care for themselves and their children can continue to build on this foundation.

The nurse's first responsibility to the pregnant woman is to be sure she is under medical supervision. The public health nurse probably has the most frequent contacts with these women, but the hospital or clinic nurse may have similar opportunities. If through casual and tactful conversation the nurse discovers that the woman is not getting prenatal care, it is important to help her to understand why she should have it and, if necessary, to suggest how she can get such care. This teaching is just as important for women who have already had children as for those who are pregnant for the first time.

In many prenatal clinics and community maternity services, organized classes are conducted on a regular and continuing basis for expectant parents. A frequent problem is that parents sometimes do not know about these classes; bulletin board announcements in hospital wards, in clinics and in medical offices, and word-of-mouth information by nurses are therefore important. Emphasis should be placed on welcoming husbands to these classes. Expectant fathers are sometimes reluctant to attend because they feel awkward about "being the only man there" or embarrassed about discussing pregnancy and delivery. Encouraging their attendance is important because these classes provide an opportunity for them to learn about pregnancy and the birth of the baby and to gain some understanding of their role as husbands and future fathers.

Nurses who teach these classes find that they can be stimulating and satisfying both to the teacher and to the learners, particularly when emphasis is placed on discussion rather than lectures and when the topics for consideration are raised by the prospective parents rather than the teacher. The parents attending these classes are usually well motivated and enjoy sharing their experiences with each other; the practitioner's chief problem seems to be to include all the topics on pregnancy, delivery, and child-rearing that the learners want to know about, in the time available.

Parents of School Children

Opportunities for teaching the parents of school children vary according to the policies of different school systems. In some schools the nurse is free to make home visits when children are ill or when there are health problems that need attention. Some schools arrange for nurse-parent conferences at the school; sometimes the nurse may be asked to participate in the teacher-parent conferences that are scheduled at regular intervals. All these contacts enable the nurse to initiate health teaching with parents, using the specific problem of the child as a starting point and later widening the area of discussion to include other family members and health problems in general.

Parent-teacher association meetings provide opportunities to contact groups of parents. Most parents are very much interested in their children's health and would welcome a discussion by the school nurse. If time is allowed in the meeting for a question period and opportunity is given for parents to talk individually with the nurse afterwards, the nurse may pick up many clues about the extent of the parents' understanding of health problems in general and specific needs for health education in certain families.

Students of Nursing

Nursing practitioners do not have a direct responsibility for teaching students of nursing; this is a function of the instructors on the nursing school faculty. However, the practitioner often works in the same area or unit where students are assigned and therefore has a most important responsibility—that of setting an example of good nursing care and appropriate professional conduct. We have discussed imitation as a way of learning. The instruction the student receives from the school faculty can be reinforced or weakened by what the student sees in actual practice. This is not an implication that the practitioner should give better nursing care or be more careful of conduct in the presence of students than when there are no students on the unit; the point is made to indicate that the practitioner has this indirect responsibility toward these students.

CO-WORKERS SUPERVISED BY THE PRACTITIONER

The nursing practitioner is responsible for teaching a variety of co-workers, including other nursing practitioners, practical nurses, nursing assistants, hospital ward clerks, office secretaries, and volunteer workers. In settings where the personnel who give nursing care are organized into nursing teams, the team leader will probably carry most of this responsibility; in other settings, all practitioners exercise this function.

Some of the factors that are likely to influence the teaching and learning of co-workers are the worker's educational background, his age and experience, and his feelings about his job security.

Educational Background

Since teaching must be based on what the learner has already had an opportunity to learn, it is important that the nurse be aware of the co-worker's previous general education and preparation in nursing. Some will have completed only elementary school; some, high school; some will have finished college. The amount of previous preparation in nursing may also show a wide range, from the volunteer worker or nursing assistant who has had very little, to the nursing practitioner who has graduated from a baccalaureate nursing program.

There are also marked differences in what co-workers with supposedly similar educational backgrounds have learned during their formal education. It is a mistake to assume, for example, that because two practical nurses have graduated from practical nurse programs, they will be equally proficient in their work or will have similar attitudes about their learning experiences. Each co-worker must be seen as an individual; what he already knows and his attitudes about both learning and nursing are important to be known before teaching is undertaken.

Age and Experience

The recently graduated nursing practitioner may find that many co-workers are older and have had much more experience than the practitioner. The mere fact of age and years of experience does not necessarily mean that these workers cannot profit from the nurse's teaching, but it does mean that in some instances they may feel resentful of the younger person's supervising their work and "telling them what to do." This resentment may be justified if the inexperienced nurse who has more education than the workers ignores what the workers may have learned in their years of nursing experience and rushes in to teach them things they already know.

The practitioner will find it worthwhile to proceed slowly, to get to know these workers and their backgrounds, to treat them with respect and courtesy, and to observe their performance in giving nursing care before making specific plans for teaching. Commending them on good work without being patronizing and seeking their help and advice when it is appropriate may dispel some of the resentment and will also enable the nurse to profit from the worker's experience.

Job Security

The worker's concern for his job, and therefore his means of livelihood, may be a factor that enters into nurse-co-worker relationships. Since the practitioner is responsible not only for teaching but also for evaluating nursing performance, some workers may feel insecure and anxious in their contacts with the nurse. This supervisory relationship is a reality that the nurse and the worker must accept, and the nurse must take it into consideration as an overt or concealed factor in dealing with co-workers.

CO-WORKERS IN SCHOOLS AND INDUSTRY

The practitioner works primarily in a cooperative relationship with teachers in schools and supervisory personnel in industry. Although schools and industry are concerned with the health of pupils and employees, their primary objectives are, respectively, education and production. Thus, the nurse has a different relationship to co-workers here than would be the case in a hospital, public health agency, or doctor's office, where the main objective is health. When the doctor is not in attendance, the nurse may be the only representative of the health professions in these settings and therefore may have the major responsibility for the health program. Cooperative relationships must be developed with teachers and with industrial supervisors so that health education may be carried on without interfering with the primary goals of these institutions. If there is good rapport and teaching aims are clarified, the nurse's plans will receive support from teachers and supervisors, and they in turn may feel free to make suggestions that will be helpful to the nurse, based on their observations of the health needs of the pupils or workers.

SUMMARY

We have discussed a variety of problems that may exist for both learners and teachers in nursing situations. The nurse will not meet all these problems with every group of learners, of course, but the possibility that these difficulties may exist in certain circumstances should not be overlooked. Each situation must be examined individually. The obvious similarities and differences in various settings or relationships are not likely to cause problems; it is the subtle, hidden factors which are not at once apparent that may cause difficulties and present a challenge to the nurse.

REFERENCES

BENDER, RUTH E. "Communicating with the Deaf." *American Journal of Nursing* 66:757-60, April, 1966.
The author, a speech and hearing expert, discusses ways of maintaining adequate communication with people who are deaf, and illustrates her points with incidents from her experience.

FOX, MADELINE J. "Talking with Patients Who Can't Answer." *American Journal of Nursing* 71:1146-49, June, 1971.
Although we have not discussed aphasia because it is such a complex area, this article will give the reader at least some idea of the enormous difficulties these patients face in learning to speak again.

GASPARD, NANCY J. "The Family of the Patient with Long-Term Illness." *Nursing Clinics of North America* 5:77-84, March, 1970.
This is a very good discussion of the reactions of both patient and family to the prospect of long-term illness and of the role of the nurse in helping all who are involved. The effect on young children is also discussed.

GRIM, ROSEMARY A. "Mr. Edwards' Triumph." *American Journal of Nursing* 72:480-81, March, 1972.
Mr. Edwards is a blind man living alone, who developed diabetes at the age of 63. With the teaching done by the public health nurse in his home,

he was able to give himself his insulin and manage his diet with minimal supervision and thus maintained his independence.

HORNER, ADA L., and JENNINGS, MURIEL. "Before Patients Go Home." *American Journal of Nursing* 61:62-63, June, 1961.
The authors describe a program for preparing family members to care for patients at home through classes and supervised care of the patient in the hospital before he is discharged.

HULICKA, IRENE M. "Fostering Self-Respect in Aging Patients." *American Journal of Nursing* 61:44-47, May, 1961.
The author shows a deep understanding of the aged patient's need for self-respect and how this need can be met by hospital nurses and nursing assistants.

JACKSON, GEORGE D. "How Blind Are Nurses to the Needs of the Visually Handicapped?" *Nursing Outlook* 13:34-37, September, 1965.
The author, a psychologist, blind since childhood, analyzes why sighted people, including nurses, have difficulty relating to blind people.

LARSEN, VIRGINIA. "What Hospitalization Means to Patients." *American Journal of Nursing* 61:44-47, May, 1961.
This article reviews the expectations, needs, and fears of hospital patients of all ages and discusses the concept of the "cooperative patient."

MUECKE, MARJORIE A. "Overcoming the Language Barrier." *Nursing Outlook* 18:53-54, April, 1970.
A brief but very good article on ways of communicating with patients who do not speak English. The article ends with a simple, effective list of suggestions for communicating with patients, regardless of their language capacity.

NILO, ERNEST R. "Needs of the Hearing Impaired." *American Journal of Nursing* 69:114-16, January, 1969.
This article deals with the need for early detection of hearing impairment, the effects and identification of such impairment, and rehabilitation programs.

NORRIS, CATHERINE M. "The Work of Getting Well." *American Journal of Nursing* 69:2118-21, October, 1969.
This is an excellent article that points out the patient's problems during convalescence and the difficulties families may have during this period.

OHNO, MARY I. "The Eye-Patched Patient." *American Journal of Nursing* 71:271-74, February, 1971.
The author presents an overall view of sensory deprivation—what it is and how it affects patients—and then shows how eye-patched patients are in this group and what can be done by teaching and by nursing measures to alleviate the problem.

PETERSON, DONALD I. "Developing the Difficult Patient." *American Journal of Nursing* 67:522-25, March, 1967.
This is a humorous article until the reader is about halfway through—then it becomes very "unfunny." The title means just what it says and shows clearly how much of a patient's "difficultness" may be caused by the care he receives.

RICHIE, JEANNE, "Using an Interpreter Effectively." *Nursing Outlook* 12:27-29, December, 1964.

The author, a public health nurse who has worked in Nigeria and South America, discusses problems in working with interpreters and suggests ways of avoiding misunderstandings.

SORENSON, KAREN M., and AMIS, DOROTHY BRUNER. "Understanding the World of the Chronically Ill." *American Journal of Nursing* 67:811-17, April, 1967. This article presents many facets of the problems of the patient who has a chronic illness and makes clear his alienation from life and, in some instances, his feelings of hopelessness.

STONE, VIRGINIA. "Give the Older Person Time." *American Journal of Nursing* 69:2124-27, October, 1969. Older people need enough time to perceive, to respond, to learn, and to move and act—the nurse who is constantly aware of this fact will make life more comfortable for older patients and have satisfaction in working with them.

SYKES, ELEANOR M., "No Time for Silence." *American Journal of Nursing* 66: 1040-41, May, 1966. Communication problems of people who cannot speak are exemplified in this discussion of the nurse's role in communicating with patients who have just had laryngectomies.

"Symposium on Patients with Sensory Defects." *Nursing Clinics of North America* 5:449-538, September, 1970. Five articles in this symposium have particular relevance for the reader; although only one article is directly concerned with teaching, all of them contribute ideas about working with patients who have some sort of sensory deprivation:

> CHODIL, JUDITH, and WILLIAMS, BARBARA. "The Concept of Sensory Deprivation," pp. 453-65.
> CONDL, EMMA D. "Ophthalmic Nursing: The Gentle Touch," pp. 467-76.
> CONOVER, MARY, and COBR, JOYCE. "Understanding and Caring for the Hearing-Impaired," pp. 497-506.
> CULLIN, IRENE C. "Techniques for Teaching Patients with Sensory Defects," pp. 527-38.
> PARVULESCU, NINA F. "Care of the Surgically Speechless Patient," pp. 517-25.

WOOD, MAXINE. *Blindness—Ability, Not Disability.* New York, Public Affairs Pamphlets, #295A, 1968. Miss Wood discusses blindness with a positive, optimistic point of view and covers a great variety of topics of interest to blind people, lay people, and the professional practitioner.

Chapter _____ *5*

The Subject Matter

The subject matter to be taught to clients and co-workers may include almost everything practitioners have learned in basic nursing programs, from the simplest facts of hygiene to the scientific principles and techniques of complex nursing care. It is not within the scope of this book to attempt to discuss the details of this content—you learn this in your nursing program and you continue to learn new content throughout your nursing career. We will be concerned here with the broad areas of subject matter that the nurse may have occasion to teach. The chapter will be divided into three sections: (1) content related to health status, (2) content related to giving nursing care, and (3) content related to the orientation of new workers. Both clients and co-workers may be taught content from either of the first two areas.

CONTENT RELATED TO HEALTH STATUS

Subject matter relating to health status includes content about the patient's current illness, convalescence, and the prevention of illness and the promotion of health.

Current Illness

You are already aware of the need for the patient, his family, and those who give him nursing care to understand the nature of the patient's illness. Before planning to teach the patient or his family, the practitioner must find out what the physician has told them and what he wants them to be taught. This is particularly true when the patient has a poor prognosis or is in the terminal stage of illness. It is the doctor's prerogative to determine what the patient and his family should be told and the nurse must be guided by his decision. There are generally no restrictions on teaching co-workers about the patient's condition.

Information about the present illness may include the causes, predisposing and precipitating factors, the usual course and duration of the illness, the doctor's plan of care and its purpose, and the objectives of nursing care. Whether all this material is taught, and the detail in which it is presented, will be determined by the learner's ability to comprehend it, and his learning needs. For example, in most situations the patient and his family do not need to be taught the details of the medical care that has been instituted, while the co-worker caring for the patient may have a need for this information; at the same time, a nursing assistant does not need to learn the complex principles underlying the patient's medical care, while a nursing practitioner who has not cared for a patient with this type of illness might very well be taught these principles. Except for the doctor's prerogative mentioned above, the practitioner usually makes the decision as to what is to be taught, and to whom, and in how much detail; these decisions must be based on a careful evaluation of each situation.

Convalescence

The primary task for convalescent patients is to give up their dependence on the nurse and to assume responsibility for themselves. Some patients can make this transition very easily, others find it very difficult. Sometimes nurses, without realizing it, derive satisfaction from having patients dependent on them and unconsciously encourage dependency by continuing to do things for the patient which he should be doing for himself. Teaching directed toward self-care and the prevention of further illness may help the patient to assume increasing responsibility for himself. If there seem to be indications that the patient is afraid he will harm himself in some way, the physical presence of the nurse and reassurance as to his safety may be helpful. At the same time the patient should not be pushed toward independence too quickly after acute illness, lest he lose confidence and stop trying to help himself.

The teaching at this time is primarily concerned with interpreting the doctor's plans for continuing therapy and making it clear to the patient how he may be able to avoid a recurrence of this illness and maintain good health. It is important, if at all possible, that the family member who will be responsible for the patient during the rest of his convalescence also be made aware of these points; hospital co-workers who will be caring for convalescing patients also need information of this kind.

The practitioner will need to check with the patient's physician to find out what continuing medical treatment will be ordered, whether the patient is to return to see the doctor at his office or at the hospital outpatient department, and if there is to be a referral to a public health nursing agency. Since the patient will be "on his own" after he is discharged from the hospital, it is important that he understand the need for any further treatment and that he be given specific instructions about further appointments to see his doctor.

The patient's family should be given some understanding of the problems the patient may have in resuming independence and must also be warned against helping him remain dependent by doing things for him that he can do for himself, or, on the other hand, letting him do too much too soon. The family should be made aware that they should consult the physician when questions arise during convalescence at home.

Teaching about the prevention of the recurrence of the illness can be easily combined with teaching about the health principles necessary for maintaining good general health. This teaching may be instituted by the hospital nurse and continued by the nurse in the clinic, the doctor's office, or the public health nursing agency.

Prevention of Illness and Promotion of Health

The practitioner may frequently have occasion to teach concepts concerning the prevention of illness and the promotion of health to clients and co-workers. Young people and adults, people who are sick and those who are well, parents and other family members, co-workers—all these groups need to understand and be able to apply health principles. A vital need of society as a whole is being met when people know how to avoid illness and maintain optimum health, whether this knowledge is applied to themselves, to their families, or to the people to whom they give nursing care or health supervision.

The content in this area includes so much that we can do no more here than indicate the general outline of what might be taught. Some of this content applies to people of all ages, some applies to people of particular age groups; this material may be taught to people in good health or may be modified to fit the learning needs of people with special health problems. Some of the areas may be summarized as follows:

1. General hygiene
   a. Personal and environmental cleanliness
   b. Nutrition and eating habits
   c. Elimination
   d. Exercise, rest, and sleep
   e. Dental hygiene
   f. Care of the eyes and ears
   g. Hygiene of menstruation
   h. Hygiene of pregnancy and the postpartum period
   i. Mental hygiene

2. Importance of physical examinations
   a. Regular medical examinations and chest x-rays
   b. Regular dental examinations
   c. Special examinations
      (1) Examination of infants and preschool children
      (2) Eye examinations and vision tests
      (3) Ear examinations and hearing tests
      (4) Prenatal and postpartum examinations
      (5) Examinations after traumatic injuries
3. Prevention of infections
   a. Care of respiratory infections
   b. Care of breaks in the skin
   c. Warning signs of local or general infections
   d. Immunizations against infectious diseases
4. Early cancer detection
   a. Symptoms of cancer
   b. Methods for early detection
   c. Responsibility of the individual for reporting suspicious symptoms
5. Prevention of accidents
   a. Fire
   b. Falls
   c. Poisoning
   d. Drowning
   e. Electric shock
   f. Injury due to poor body mechanics
   g. Supervision of small children

CONTENT RELATED TO GIVING NURSING CARE

Subject matter relating to giving nursing care includes content about general supportive nursing care and the performance of nursing procedures.

General Supportive Nursing Care

There will be many opportunities to teach both nursing co-workers in health agencies and family members at home about the principles of general nursing care and meeting the needs of people who are ill. Perhaps one of the most important concepts for the person who is giving nursing care to understand about sick people is that, in general, their needs are the same as those of people in good health, but that these needs may have to be met differently. One difference lies in the fact that patients are often unable to meet their needs themselves and this responsibility therefore falls entirely on those who are giving nursing care.

Another difference is that the ways of meeting these needs may have to be modified and adapted because of the patient's physical condition, as, for example, whether he is confined to bed, his state of consciousness, the extent to which he is able and willing to help, and, in some cases, whether the doctor will allow him to help himself. If the person who is giving nursing care knows how to give supportive care to a helpless bed patient, there should be little difficulty in making adaptations for patients who are less dependent.

By general supportive nursing care, we mean providing for the patient's hygienic needs and comfort, regardless of the nature of the illness. Teaching will relate to such specific areas as cleanliness of the patient's person and his environment, adequate rest and sleep, proper nutrition and elimination, protection of the skin from irritation and pressure, proper body alignment and regular change of position, as well as attention to the patient's safety and emotional well-being.

When a family member is being taught to give nursing care in the home, several additional points might be included. It will be helpful if the nurse discusses the adaptation of available furniture and household equipment for the comfort of the patient and the convenience of the person who is giving the care. For example, back rests, bedside tables, and trays for serving meals can be easily improvised; raising the bed on sturdy wooden blocks will make it easier to give care to patients who must remain in bed; adequate protection of the furniture in the sick room will prevent damage and make cleaning easier. The nurse should also make suggestions as to how plans can be made for giving care to the patient with the least amount of interruption to the household and to family activities—it is important that the needs of all of the family be given consideration during the patient's illness at home.

Performance of Nursing Procedures

The nursing procedures that the practitioner may teach are too numerous to be itemized here, but we can specify certain basic information that should be taught about procedures in general. The person who is giving nursing care should know the reasons for doing a procedure, how to perform it safely and effectively, and the expected therapeutic result. Knowing these things, the person giving the care will be able to perform the procedure more efficiently, evaluate its therapeutic effectiveness, and, when necessary, make safe and appropriate modifications to meet various patients' needs.

Teaching about procedures should include a discussion of the equipment that is needed, the physical and psychological preparation of the patient, written or oral reporting of the results of the treatment to the doctor or nurse, and aftercare of the patient, the unit, and the equipment that has been used.

Since so many nursing procedures are prescribed by the physician, emphasis must be placed on teaching the importance of careful checking of orders to determine exactly what is to be done and how often, the strength and temperature of solutions to be used, when the procedure is to be discontinued, and so forth.

Co-workers in busy hospital wards and clinics should be taught to be aware of the necessity for accurate identification of patients before procedures are started, preferably by asking the patient to state his full name or checking the identification arm band if there is one. This is particularly important when several patients in the unit have the same last name, when the patient does not speak English, or where there are many patients out of bed and moving freely about the unit.

CONTENT RELATED TO THE ORIENTATION OF NEW WORKERS

Orientation of new workers to the nursing unit is an important process, not only for the effective functioning of the unit, but also for the personal adjustment and work satisfaction of the new employee. If the agency has an inservice orientation program, the nurse will probably have no formal responsibility in this area, but in any situation the nurse will have an informal responsibility to make the worker feel welcome and help him learn about the specific details of the particular unit to which he has been assigned. If he has had a general orientation to the agency, the nurse should know what has been discussed in order to avoid repetitions and omissions in his orientation to the unit.

Of primary importance to the worker is the development of a feeling of belonging in this new setting. The nurse can be instrumental in bringing this about by greeting him in a friendly way, by introducing him to other co-workers, and by making a definite effort to include him in the activities of the unit. The worker who feels truly welcome is likely to adjust more easily and function more effectively in his new position than the worker who feels like the fifth wheel on a wagon.

Early in his orientation the worker will need to know about such things as the scheduling of working hours and meals, locker and dressing facilities, the procedure for reporting on and off duty, when and where he will be paid, and to whom he is directly responsible for his work.

At appropriate times, the worker should be taught the policies and routines of the hospital and of the unit where he is working, the standards of performance that are expected, and how and when his work will be evaluated. The nurse should anticipate that the worker may not remember everything that has been explained and should expect that there will have to be a certain amount of repetition, as in any teaching-learning situation. If a comfortable relationship has been developed, the worker will probably feel free to ask the nurse about things he has forgotten or does not understand.

The effective orientation of new workers can contribute directly to the smooth operation of the nursing unit, to the job satisfaction of the worker, and to the quality of care being given by the nursing personnel.

SUMMARY

The material presented in this chapter has provided only a broad outline of the kinds of subject matter the practitioner may teach to clients and co-workers. In determining the details of content to be taught to each learner, the nurse will have to call upon knowledge gained as a student of nursing and, later, as a graduate nurse, and keep up to date on new information by making a habit of reading current books and journals in nursing and other related fields.

The reference readings for this chapter include several articles concerned with patients who have particular health problems. These articles have been selected as examples of ways of organizing content in planning teaching; there is no implication intended that these topics are any more important than the numerous other subjects the practitioner may have occasion to teach.

REFERENCES

BURNSIDE, IRENE MORTENSON. "Things My Nursing Instructor Never Taught Me!" *Nursing Outlook* 11:124-25, February, 1963.
This article, written with appropriate humor, gives an account of how a public health nurse learned to improvise in the home.

CHERESCAVICH, GERTRUDE D. A *Textbook for Nursing Assistants,* 2d ed. St. Louis: C. V. Mosby Company, 1968.
This textbook presents details of the content that may be taught to nursing assistants.

HAMMOND, EDITH. "Home Care and Improvisations."*Nursing Outlook* 12:49-51. April, 1964.
This article, which is focused on the home care of the patient with cancer, will be of value to the practitioner in teaching any type of patient in the home.

HOEPER, BEATRICE. "A Lesson in Positive Health." *Nursing Outlook* 8:614-15, November, 1960.
This article describes the expansion of an industrial health program from a "first-aid" point of view to a concept of broad health education for employees.

KRYSAN, GERMAINE S. "How Do We Teach Four Million Diabetics?" *American Journal of Nursing* 65:105-7, November, 1965.
The author, a Public Health Service consultant, reviews the learning needs of our diabetic population and suggests ways for coordinating teaching and follow-up in the community.

LINEHAN, DOROTHY T. "What Does the Patient Want to Know?" *American Journal of Nursing* 66:1066-70, May, 1966.
This is a report of a study of what hospital patients want to know upon discharge. Among other recommendations, plans for more and improved patient teaching are discussed.

SCHLOTTER, LOWANNA. "Learning to Be a Home Dialysis Patient—Trials and Tribulations." *Nursing Clinics of North America* 4:419-29, September, 1969.
This article emphasizes the patient's problems in adjusting to complex care at home. The author discusses applications of principles of learning and teaching and shows great sensitivity to the patient.

SESSOMS, DEEDA. "A Safety Project in Elementary School." *American Journal of Nursing* 60:1288-89, September, 1960.
This article describes how the school nurse and the teachers in a public school cooperated in developing an effective safety project for fifth- and sixth-grade pupils.

WEAVER, BARBARA, and WILLIAMS, ELSIE L. "Teaching the Tuberculosis Patient." *American Journal of Nursing* 63:80-82, December, 1963.
The authors describe a successful teaching program for hospital patients, including content, methods, and materials, and the application of principles of learning and teaching.

Chapter _____ 6

Methods of Teaching

The methods of teaching that the practitioner will find most appropriate in nursing situations are those that are generally used in more or less informal settings with one learner at a time or with small groups of learners. We will limit our discussion to such methods. Formal classroom instruction with large groups is not usually part of the practitioner's teaching function; nurses who do have this kind of responsibility should have more advanced preparation for teaching than is encompassed in this book.

The methods of teaching to be considered in this chapter will be discussed under the following headings: (1) informal teaching, (2) structured teaching, and (3) teaching through supervision.

INFORMAL TEACHING

By informal teaching we mean here the somewhat casual unstructured teaching that may take place in almost every contact the nurse has with clients or co-workers. This kind of teaching may be "on-the-spot" teaching, as when the learner asks a question that shows a need for teaching; it may sometimes be initiated by the nurse to meet a learning need that has been identified; it may take place without the actual awareness of either nurse or learner, as when a client or co-worker adopts an attitude or a habit by observing the nurse's behavior. The fact that the words *casual* and *unstructured* are used to describe this kind of teaching must not be interpreted as meaning unimportant or offhand. Informal teaching constitutes a large part of the practitioner's teaching and accounts for an important part of the learning of clients and co-workers. It may include talking and listening, asking and answering questions, and setting an example.

Talking and Listening

Talking and listening as techniques in informal teaching are something more than the casual and friendly give-and-take of social conversation. When we chat with friends or acquaintances, we may talk without any particular direction or any purpose other than sociability. We are sometimes more interested in what we have to contribute than in listening to what the other person is saying. A certain amount of this kind of conversation with clients or co-workers may serve to establish a comfortable climate and may inadvertently give clues to the nurse about learning needs, but if the practitioner's teaching objectives are to be realized, random conversation and listening with "half an ear" must be replaced by purposeful talking and effective listening.

By purposeful talking we mean communicating with the learner with a definite goal in mind. In early contacts with patients and their families, the goals might be to determine their feelings about the patient's illness, their understanding and acceptance of the medical therapy and nursing care the patient is receiving, and something about their family relationships. Similarly, talking with a purpose to co-workers may reveal their attitudes about nursing, their feelings about their competence in giving nursing care, and their relationships to patients and to other co-workers. Thus, purposeful talking lays the groundwork for further teaching.

By effective listening we mean actually receiving and correctly interpreting what is being communicated. Many people seem to think they are listening simply by virtue of the fact that they are quiet when someone else is talking. This may be an indication of good manners, but it is not listening. Listening is an active process which requires close attention to what is being said and how it is being said. It requires that we use not only our ears to hear the words that are being spoken, but also our eyes to observe facial expressions and gestures, and our minds to be aware of what is *not* being said as well as what *is* being said. Sometimes there is a great disparity between what someone says and what he means; often what is being concealed is more significant than what is being said. Avoidance of a topic we might expect a learner to mention, as, for example, his impending surgery, may mean that he is unable at this point to face the problem by himself and needs help to express his difficulties openly. On the other hand, another patient who does not talk about his impending surgery may have no need to, and may thus prefer to talk about other things. The point here is that the practitioner must be sensitive to patients' reactions, helping the patient who wants to talk about his concerns, and respecting the rights of the patient who does not. Effective listening is thus an important tool in teaching and the nurse will find that the development of this skill requires practice in the same way as do other nursing skills.

Asking and Answering Questions

Another technique of informal teaching consists in asking and answering questions. Just as with talking and listening, we are concerned here with a purposeful process—questions asked and answers given with the needs of the learner in mind in order to fulfill our teaching objectives.

Merely to ask questions is not difficult; think of some youngster you know and reflect on the ease with which he may ask dozens of questions every day. Asking significant questions in a way that is acceptable to the learner, however, is quite a different matter. Many of the questions a nurse will want to ask to determine learning needs are of a personal nature. Learners may resent such questions if they are asked before some measure of rapport has been built up or if they are asked in such a way that they give the impression of prying into personal matters. If the nurse has established a good relationship with the learner and he sees that answering such questions will be of benefit to him, he is quite likely to respond. If, on the other hand, questions are asked as if the nurse had a perfect right to ask them and to expect an answer regardless of the learner's feeling about replying, the learner is likely to refuse to answer or to become evasive and hostile. It is probable that very few nurses use a "third-degree" technique with patients or their families, but, unfortunately, there are some nurses who do seem to think they have a right to use this method, particularly with the co-workers they supervise. This kind of questioning not only fails to accomplish its real purpose, but may also set up insurmountable barriers to any cooperative effort toward teaching and learning.

Another aspect of effective questioning is the nurse's response to the answers that are given to the questions. Unless there is some strong evidence to the contrary, the nurse should assume that the patient has answered to the best of his ability, no matter how inaccurate or surprising the answer may be. Remarks, facial expressions, or gestures on the part of the nurse that indicate disbelief, amazement, or ridicule will embarrass or antagonize the learner and may result in his refusal to answer any further questions. The nurse who matter-of-factly accepts whatever answer is given will be able to maintain a channel of communication with the learner and at the same time evaluate the response in relation to his learning needs.

Lastly, the questions asked by the learner may have a direct bearing on the practitioner's teaching. It is important to remember that there is a purpose behind the questions people ask. Sometimes the reason is obvious: to get information, to start a conversation, or merely to say something. Sometimes the reason may be obscure, as when someone asks an indirect question to get reassurance or to broach a topic he is afraid to approach directly. The nurse who is alert to the possibility that the motive behind the question may be hidden even from the learner will not make the error of categorizing it as a "foolish" question and giving a superficial answer. Exploring the possible reasons behind questions can give the nurse valuable insights into some of the learner's problems.

Setting an Example

In the chapter on the principles of learning, we discussed the importance of imitation as a method of learning. In nursing situations the practitioner is continually setting an example for the learner, consciously or unconsciously, and the learner is continually either accepting or rejecting the example, consciously or unconsciously. When teaching and learning by example are conscious processes, the situation can be controlled and evaluated; it is possible to determine specific learning outcomes. When the process is on an unconscious level, the practitioner will probably never really know what has been learned.

A large part of the learning that results from the example set by the nurse concerns attitudes—attitudes about health and illness, attitudes about nurses and nursing, attitudes about doctors and the therapy they prescribe. This process goes on in any situation in which the practitioner is identified as a nurse: in the hospital, in the clinic, in the home, and even in settings completely removed from nursing. People form their opinions (and their stereotypes) about nurses and nursing from the nurses they see, and their judgments are based on the nurse's behavior. Thus, teaching by setting a favorable example can have far-reaching effects, both on those people for whom the nurse has a direct nursing responsibility and on the general public.

STRUCTURED TEACHING

When we speak here of structured teaching, we are referring to instruction that is planned in advance according to a definite teaching guide or outline and scheduled for a specific time and place for one or several learners. In planning and carrying out structured teaching, the techniques of informal teaching (talking, questioning, setting an example) are also used, but with the difference that they are deliberately planned beforehand. For example, the nurse will work out the opening remarks that will be used to introduce the topic, prepare questions to be asked during the lesson, and plan for setting an example of the appropriate attitudes or behavior during the class.

In a later chapter we will discuss how to develop a plan for structured teaching. In this chapter we will be concerned with two methods of structured teaching that are appropriate for the practitioner's teaching in nursing settings: discussion and demonstration.

Discussion Method

Discussion is a method of teaching in which a small group of learners and the teacher talk about a particular topic in an informal way. In a productive discussion, it is usually the learners who are active, while the teacher stays more or less in the background. Probably the chief factor that makes for a worthwhile discussion is the knowledge and experience the learners already have about the subject. At the first meeting (or during the first few minutes if there is to be only one meeting), some time will have to be devoted to undirected discussion, simply to find out what the learners know about the topic and what their learning needs may be. There are few more effective ways to waste time and produce boredom in the learners (and the teacher, as well) than having a discussion that is merely a sharing of ignorance. The little time that is usually available for the nurse's teaching is too precious to be wasted in this way. If the discussions can be scheduled in advance and the participants notified of the topic, the nurse will be able to plan the teaching more effectively, and the learners will have an opportunity to think about the subject beforehand.

Discussion as a method of teaching is best suited to a rather small group of learners, although some of the principles presented here may be used with larger groups or with an individual. Probably the optimum size group would be from six to ten people. With fewer people there may not be a great enough variety of ideas contributed to sustain a stimulating discussion; with a larger group, the participation of everyone will be impossible.

Opportunities for using this method of teaching may exist wherever small groups of learners with similar learning needs can be assembled; for example, the up-patients or the nursing personnel in a hospital unit, the patients waiting for clinic or office appointments, the parents visiting schools for parent-teacher meetings or "open house" days.

Teaching people in groups has several advantages. When the members of a group become aware that they have similar problems and when they feel free to discuss these problems and raise questions of mutual concern, participation of everyone in the group may be stimulated. A question asked by one person may be of interest to many others, and less vocal members may be encouraged to voice their opinions. The sharing of ideas and experiences focused on common problems offers benefits to the learners that are not possible in teaching individual learners. It is obvious that there is also an advantage to the nurse in the time saved when several individuals can be taught at once. It is also important to include here the advantage to the nurse in the stimulation offered to the teacher as well as the learner in a lively, productive discussion. Whether or not these advantages are realized depends largely on the relationships within the group and the general climate of the learning setting; the practitioner can be instrumental in influencing both of these factors.

Let us assume that the nurse has arranged for a discussion with a group of patients who are meeting together for the first time. Since we are concerned at this point with the techniques of discussion rather than the content, we will also assume that the nurse has already planned the subject matter for the class and is about to make final preparations.

The room to be used for the meeting should be checked far enough in advance to assure that it will be ready when the group assembles. When the physical setting is comfortable and in good order, the learner's first impression will be favorable; it may help to make him more at ease and encourage him to return again. His attitudes in this respect are particularly important, since he is usually present voluntarily and it is entirely up to him whether he returns. Among the things that should be checked in the room are cleanliness, lighting, ventilation, temperature, and seating space.

The arrangement of chairs for group discussion deserves special mention. If at all possible, the seats should be arranged in an informal circle in which the nurse is included. This will make it possible for everyone to see and hear each other and will encourage communication among members of the group. When the nurse is behind a desk at the front of the room and the learners are lined up in straight rows, the nurse cannot help but become the center of attention and, in a sense, an authority figure; questions and comments will usually be directed solely to the teacher and any real discussion among the group members will be less likely. Under these conditions, the whole purpose of group discussion as a method of teaching may be thwarted simply because of the inappropriate seating arrangements.

The nurse should be in the room before the scheduled time for the discussion to greet people when they arrive and to make introductions. Time will be well spent if the nurse tries to learn the members' names and use them as soon as possible, thus giving recognition to each learner and helping the group members to get acquainted. Inviting people to take off their coats and hats and sit down where they wish will help to make them feel welcome; if anyone seems to be ill at ease, a little extra effort by the nurse may make him feel more comfortable. The class should be started as promptly as possible in order not to waste time, but late arrivals should be made to feel welcome.

In the first meeting of a new group, it is the nurse's responsibility to take the initiative by discussing the purpose of the class and giving some sort of introduction to the topic. This will give the members of the group an opportunity to adjust themselves to the situation and begin to feel comfortable. As questions for discussion are introduced, they should be very general and related to areas that the learners are sure to have information about, so that they will feel confident in answering. It is best to ask these introductory questions of the group as a whole so that no one feels he is being put "on a spot" in front of the others. As the class proceeds, the questions may become more specific. If the nurse knows something about the background of some of the members, they may be encouraged to talk about their particular experience in relation to the topic.

As the group begins to take some initiative in the discussion, the role of the nurse may shift from active participant to active listener and observer. The responsibility now becomes a matter of keeping the group on the topic, tactfully correcting errors or misunderstandings, and encouraging everyone to take part. In almost any group there will be those who talk easily and those who tend to be less vocal. It is up to the nurse to be sure that everyone has a chance to participate. It is also up to the nurse to be aware of the reactions of the group members which indicate that there is a need for clarification or further discussion on some particular point. The nurse's constant attention is necessary during group discussion.

At the end of the discussion there should be a summary of what has been said and a review of the major points that have been covered. It is helpful to the nurse in evaluating the effectiveness of the discussion to have group members summarize what they think are the important ideas they got from the class. Sometimes, however, as with a new group or when time is short, the nurse may present the summary. If the group is to meet again, the time and place of the next meeting and the topic to be discussed should be announced.

Directly after the discussion is concluded, the nurse will find it profitable to review the dynamics of the session and try to determine how the techniques might be improved in future sessions. These are some of the questions which might be considered: Did I give enough direction so that the purposes of the discussion were accomplished? Did all the members seem to feel comfortable in the situation? Was I able to include everyone in the discussion and did all members have a chance to speak when they wanted to? Did the group members become really interested and involved in the topic and make worthwhile contributions? If this was not the case, what can I do in future discussions to improve the way I use this method of teaching?

Demonstration Method

Demonstration is a method of teaching skills and techniques related to nursing care that can be used with equal effectiveness for both individual and group teaching. It can be employed in the hospital, the clinic, the office, or the home as long as the necessary equipment is on hand and there is adequate space available. Properly used, it is a method that is easily comprehended by the learner; if necessary, demonstrations can be conducted with very few words and therefore are especially valuable in working with learners who have a language difficulty.

The demonstration method of teaching actually has three parts: the teacher's demonstration of the technique or procedure, then supervised practice, and, lastly, the learner's return demonstration. All these steps must be included if the learner is to master the skill he is expected to learn. We will discuss the principles and techniques of each of the steps in sequence and make applications to the teaching of both individuals and groups.

A skillful demonstration requires advance preparation and practice by the teacher. Being able to perform a nursing procedure expertly in giving nursing care does not mean necessarily that the nurse will be equally expert in demonstrating the procedure to a client or co-worker. Certain modifications are required and must be practiced by the teacher if the learner is to benefit from the demonstration.

How does a demonstration differ from performing the procedure for a patient? An important difference lies in the fact that the experienced practitioner is familiar with the equipment used in the procedure and therefore handles it more or less automatically; it is easy to overlook the fact that the learners may have had no such experience and may be quite mystified by what the nurse is doing. For example, consider such a "simple" thing as a clamp on an irrigation tube. When an irrigation is being given to a patient, the nurse opens and closes the clamp without even thinking about how it is done; in a demonstration, the nurse must show the learner the clamp, explain how to open and close it, and let him try it for himself.

Another difference between performance and demonstration is in the time involved. Giving a bed bath to a patient, for example, may take about fifteen minutes; demonstrating a bed bath to a co-worker may take three-quarters of an hour or more. The demonstration must be done slowly so that the learner may see exactly what is being done and time must be allowed for explanations and questions.

A third factor that differentiates performance from demonstration is the psychological effect of self-consciousness on the nurse. It is one thing to perform expert nursing care as a familiar and established part of nursing practice; it is quite another thing to demonstrate this same care with one or several people watching every move that is made and asking questions about how and why the procedure is done in a certain way. The situation is analogous to the story of the centipede who was asked how he managed to walk with so many legs to keep track of, and when he thought about it, he became so confused that he couldn't walk at all. As the practitioner becomes accustomed to having an audience watch demonstrations, this self-consciousness will gradually disappear, but it is a factor that must be considered as this method of teaching is being perfected.

Demonstrations that are carried out for a group of learners in a classroom or ward conference room require one other modification. When nursing care is being given to a patient, the nurse may work in any position that is comfortable in relation to the patient and the equipment. When care is being demonstrated to a group seated in a classroom, the nurse may have to assume a somewhat awkward or unfamiliar position in order that the people watching may clearly see everything that is being done. As an example, a right-handed nurse may have to do some part of the demonstration with the left hand to avoid getting between the audience and the patient or the model being used to represent a patient. It may be advisable to practice working in this position before attempting it before a group. This problem is not likely to arise when demonstrating for one or two learners since they can readily change their positions in order to see.

It should now be apparent why the nurse must plan and practice in advance in order to perform a skillful demonstration. The preparation should include the following steps: (1) reviewing the purposes and steps of the procedure, (2) assembling and organizing the necessary equipment, (3) performing each step in sequence while analyzing what knowledge and skills are involved, (4) determining at what points explanations will be necessary, and (5) judging the proper speed for carrying out the demonstration and the best position for the nurse to assume in relation to the audience. It is helpful to have someone observe this practice demonstration and make suggestions for improvement, if necessary.

In preparation for the actual demonstration, the room should be checked as we have previously described, except that, for this type of class, the chairs should be arranged in whatever way is best for the learners to see and hear the teacher. Equipment should be assembled, checked to see that every piece is complete and in working order, and arranged conveniently in the order in which it will be used. If the procedure is to be demonstrated in the patient's home, the nurse should plan ahead of time with the family for any household equipment that will be needed so that it can be gotten ready beforehand.

The demonstration should be introduced by an explanation of the procedure, its purpose, and expected effects. The equipment should be shown and named, and opportunity provided for the learners to examine and handle unfamiliar items. Learners should be allowed to ask questions during the demonstration; if questions requiring lengthy discussion are asked, they should probably be held until after the procedure has been completed. During the demonstration any questions or reactions that may indicate misunderstanding or confusion should be noted and cleared up at some time during the class. If the nurse finds that the same points of confusion occur when the demonstration is given to other groups, it would be wise to try to determine whether the nurse is doing something in the demonstration that should be corrected or whether further explanation is needed, either before the demonstration is started or at the point where the learners seem to become confused. The demonstration should always include how to make the patient comfortable after the procedure is finished, how to clean the equipment, and, when it is relevant, how to record and report what has been done and the effectiveness of the treatment. It is essential that the demonstration be an example of a finished piece of work.

It is to be hoped that the practitioner will make every effort to demonstrate procedures exactly as they should be done, but if an error is made, it should be brought to the learners' attention and corrected as soon as it is discovered. At this point we might comment about teachers' errors, regardless of the method of teaching being used. Many inexperienced teachers (and even some experienced ones) refuse to admit that they have made a mistake or that they do not know the answer to every question asked of them. Perhaps they think that to admit any imperfection will somehow lower them in the learners' estimation. Actually, people are likely to admire someone who will honestly admit an error; it is the teacher who tries to cover up mistakes or lack of knowledge who falls down in the learners' opinion. However, aside from what the learners might think of the teacher, the essential point is that the teacher is responsible for giving correct information and therefore errors must be corrected.

The second part of the demonstration method of teaching is supervised practice. The amount of practice needed will depend on the complexity of the procedure, the general ability and manual skill of the learner and what experience he has had with similar procedures. As with any kind of learning, the factor that perhaps overrides all the others is the attitude of the learner—whether he sees a reason for learning that has meaning for *him*. In some instances it is possible that the learner will master the technique with very little practice; sometimes a great deal of repetition will be necessary. We have specified that practice be supervised; if the nurse can be present during the practice period, the errors that may occur can be corrected promptly and any misunderstandings can be cleared up immediately. If it is not possible for the nurse to be present, as sometimes happens, the practice will have to involve trial-and-error to some extent, and the learning will take longer and be more difficult in many cases. However, no practice should ever be permitted on an actual patient unless the nurse is present and there is no possible question of the safety of the patient.

The return demonstration is the final step of the demonstration method of teaching. After the learner has been given the opportunity to practice and feels confident of his ability to perform the procedure, he should carry out the complete procedure from start to finish, assembling the equipment, going through all the steps of the procedure, and cleaning and replacing the equipment used. If no patient is involved, the nurse should let the learner perform without interruption to be sure he can do it by himself. If the nurse gives him cues or suggestions as he works, there will be no guarantee that he can perform independently. If mistakes are made or the nurse feels any doubt about whether he can function safely, there should be further practice and another return demonstration. The nurse who is responsible for teaching is also responsible for the safe practice of the learners who have been taught.

When the teaching has been completed, the practitioner should review both the teaching that was done and the learners' responses. Some relevant questions that might be asked are these: Could my performance have been improved? Was I sure of myself in doing the procedure; was the timing right; were the learners able to see and hear what was going on; did they seem to understand the demonstration and the discussion? How well did the members of the group learn? Were they reasonably confident in handling the equipment; were they aware of the purpose and expected effects of the treatment; did they have enough opportunity for practice; were they able to perform the procedure adequately? When I do this demonstration again, what changes should I make, if any?

TEACHING THROUGH SUPERVISION

The supervisory function of the nursing practitioner is a process by which an expert practitioner guides and directs the performance of a less expert worker in order to help him improve his practice and find satisfaction in his work, with the ultimate purpose of achieving and maintaining excellent care for the patient. Supervision is inextricably bound up with teaching; in fact, a large part of effective supervision *is* teaching.

Supervision is made more effective by (1) a cooperative relationship between practitioner and co-worker, (2) knowledge about the work and the worker, (3) skillful observation, and (4) constructive evaluation. These factors will be discussed in the following sections of this chapter.

Supervision as a Cooperative Relationship

The practitioner who has supervisory responsibility for nursing personnel will find that cooperation is enhanced when there is mutual respect, an understanding by the worker of the nurse's philosophy of supervision, and a free channel of communication in both directions between the practitioner and the worker.

Mutual respect develops between the nurse and the worker when each recognizes the value of the other as an individual and as a person working toward the goal of good nursing care. The worker can respect the nurse as an expert practitioner and as a teacher who shares knowledge and skill with him to bring about excellence in patient care. The nurse can respect the worker for giving the best care of which he is capable, for his efforts to learn, and for his attempts to improve his work. In situations where the worker does not seem to be doing the best work of which he is capable, the nurse as a teacher and supervisor must accept the responsibility of making every effort to analyze the difficulty and try to correct it.

If the worker is to receive the full benefits of supervision, he must understand its purposes. Unfortunately, many of us, auxiliary workers and practitioners alike, because of our past experiences, look upon the supervisory process as authority from above focused on giving orders and criticizing mistakes, rather than as a cooperative activity intended to help us improve our performance. Such attitudes cannot be changed quickly. A certain amount of understanding can be reached by discussion with the worker, but real acceptance of the practitioner's philosophy of supervision will develop only if the worker sees objective evidence of this point of view in the practitioner's behavior. Thus, whether the worker is able to respond cooperatively to supervision depends largely on the consistent efforts of the nurse to demonstrate good supervisory practices.

Another essential factor in cooperative supervision is two-way communication between the nurse and the co-worker. We have already discussed the problems of clear communication from the practitioner's point of view. From the co-worker's point of view, some of the factors that may interfere with his communications with the nurse may be fear of authority, inability to express himself easily, reluctance to take up the nurse's time, and doubt as to how his comments or questions will be received. The nurse who takes time to talk to the worker, who helps him express his ideas, and who accepts what he has to say, will be encouraging him to communicate. Better two-way communication will solve many small problems before they can become major difficulties and, in addition, will help the nurse to evaluate the worker's performance and assess his learning needs. From the worker's viewpoint, if he is comfortable in talking with the nurse and knows that the nurse will pay attention and respond helpfully to what he says, he will be able to co-operate better in the supervisory relationship.

Knowledge About the Work and the Worker

The practitioner who is to assume the supervisory responsibility for auxiliary workers must have certain knowledge about the work to be assigned and about the nursing personnel who are to carry out the assignments.

It is assumed that the nurse who is responsible for supervising other people's work has a thorough grasp of the general objectives of nursing, understands and can apply the principles of good nursing care, and is able to perform the nursing activities assigned to co-workers. In addition, the nurse must know the policies and procedures specified by this particular agency for administering nursing care; there are many effective ways of giving patient care, but each agency establishes standards and techniques to be adhered to by its personnel.

The nurse must also know the specific job descriptions for the various categories of nursing personnel and other workers on the unit for whose work the nurse is responsible. For example, what procedures are practical nurses and nursing assistants permitted to do in this agency? What are the functions of ward clerks in this hospital? What are the duties of the secretary in this medical office? It is not enough to have just a general idea of what these workers usually do in most agencies; the nurse must know exactly what each type of worker is expected to do in this particular agency.

We have previously discussed the effect of education and nursing experience in job performance and the learning needs of co-workers. Suffice it to say here that supervision must be based on specific knowledge of each worker's background and, as far as possible, his individual potentialities.

When the nurse is thoroughly familiar with the work to be done, what kinds of work are to be assigned to each category of personnel, and something of the background that each worker brings to the job, it is possible to establish realistic standards of performance. General standards of nursing care are of course set up by the agency and the nurse in charge of the unit is responsible for seeing that these standards are maintained, but within this framework the practitioner must be sure that each worker is performing to the best of his ability and that the quality of the care he gives meets these standards.

Skillful Observation

Assessing the quality of the worker's performance depends on skillful observation by the practitioner. Observations must be frequent enough and carried out in such a way that a fair evaluation can be made.

A common problem is the tension that the worker may feel when he is being observed. Since he may not be able to do his best work under such conditions, it is important to try to relieve this anxiety. One way to accomplish this is to build up a comfortable relationship with the worker so that he looks upon the nurse as a co-worker rather than an authority figure, as a person who is observing him to help him, not just to find fault with his work. Another way to relieve this tension is to make the process of observation a regular, routine activity of the work on the unit, rather than a "special occasion." The worker who is accustomed to being observed, who has seen evidence that these observations are helpful to him, and who feels comfortable with the practitioner will not be as likely to be apprehensive. As a result he may be able to perform better and will be more likely to feel that the nurse's evaluation of his work is fair.

Another method of helping the worker to adjust to being observed and evaluated is for the nurse to work directly with him as he gives care or to work in the same room to which the worker has been assigned. This may be particularly helpful to new and inexperienced personnel or workers who seem to be especially apprehensive when they are being observed. Unless this extreme apprehension is alleviated, the purposes of the practitioner's supervision may be frustrated; excessive nervous tension is not conducive to doing good work or to learning.

There are many aspects of the worker's performance that may be noted during observations: his general approach to the patient; his understanding of the patient's physical and emotional problems; his concern for the patient's safety, comfort, and privacy; his ability to explain what he is doing for the patient and why it is being done; his technical skill in performing nursing care and attention to the details necessary for a complete piece of work.

Some observations can be made indirectly, after the care has been given. The nurse can learn a good deal about the quality of the care that has been given by observing the patient's reactions after his care, the appearance of the patient's unit, by the condition of the equipment the worker has used, and by the significance of the items the worker includes when he reports and records the care he has given.

It is usually not wise to ask the patient directly what he thinks of the care he has received. The fact that you are "the teacher" may put him almost automatically on the side of the worker and therefore he will say only positive things. On the other hand, he may be very negative for some reason. In either case such evaluations are not objective and are sometimes quite unfair to the worker. Another reason for not discussing the worker's performance with the patient is the negative effect such action may have on the patient-worker relationship or on the practitioner-worker relationship. It is the nurse who is best qualified and in the best position to evaluate the worker—it is the nurse who must accept this responsibility.

Informal teaching during observations may be very effective because the actual situation at hand provides opportunities for the learner to see the application of principles of nursing care. However, the nurse must use discretion about the teaching that is done at the patient's bedside. Most important, the patient must not get the impression that the worker is not competent and the worker must not be made to feel that the patient will no longer have confidence in him. When errors are made and corrections are necessary, they should be discussed away from the patient. There is, of course, an exception to this rule: if the worker is about to do something that will be injurious to the patient, the nurse must intervene. Even in such an event, however, it may be possible for the nurse to step in unobtrusively by saying, "Perhaps I can help you with that," or "Do you think you might do it this way?" rather than making it obvious to the patient that the worker has made or is about to make an error.

If it will not be possible for the practitioner to discuss the worker's performance with him immediately after the observation, it is important to make brief notes of what occurred and what the nurse wants to discuss. It is essential that the good points as well as what needs to be improved be noted and discussed as soon as possible, preferably while the events are fresh in the minds of both the co-worker and the practitioner.

Constructive Evaluation

Constructive evaluation was mentioned as an important component of teaching through supervision. This area will be discussed in detail in the chapter on evaluation, later in the book.

SUMMARY

This chapter has been concerned with methods of teaching appropriate to the nursing practitioner in working with clients and co-workers. Although these methods have been presented as separate techniques, they may often be used most effectively in various combinations, as when one session consists of a discussion followed by a demonstration. The nurse will probably already have developed skill in some of the aspects of the methods discussed; others will require practice and experience. The effective use of appropriate teaching techniques based on a thorough understanding of the principles of learning and teaching is important in helping people to learn.

REFERENCES

AMEND, EDITH L. "A Parent Education Program in a Children's Hospital." *Nursing Outlook* 14:53-56, April, 1966.
The author describes the cooperative efforts of a nursing staff to meet the learning needs of parents of hospitalized children. Objectives, methods, and materials are discussed.

BURKHARDT, MARTI. "Response to Anxiety." *American Journal of Nursing* 69: 2153-54, October, 1969.
The author discusses the nurse's response to patients' anxiety and suggests the simple skills of learning to listen, to be silent, to be patient and honest, and not to return anger for anger.

COYE, DOROTHY H. "Programmed Instruction for Staff Education." *American Journal of Nursing* 69:325-27, February, 1969.
Four inservice educators in a hospital employing 1500 nursing personnel set up and successfully used programmed instruction. They concluded that the time and energy needed to prepare a program necessitates careful selection of only essential and appropriate topics.

HURD, GEORGINA GREEN. "Teaching the Hemiplegic Self-Care." *American Journal of Nursing* 62:64-68, September, 1962.
The author presents a detailed discussion of the demonstration method of teaching, using a four-step method of teaching manual skills in industry for the teaching of patients.

KRON, THORA. "Nurses' Aides Need Clearer Directions." *American Journal of Nursing* 63:118-19, March, 1963.
This article discusses the practitioner's responsibility for teaching and supervising nurses' aides and emphasizes the need for giving directions in language the aide can understand.

LEFSON, ELEANOR E. "One Week's Training for the Home Health Aide." *Nursing Outlook* 14:48-50, June, 1966.
The author describes a training program for a relatively new worker, the home health aide, who functions in the home under the supervision of the public health nurse.

MEZZANOTTE, ELIZABETH JANE. "Group Instruction in Preparation for Surgery." *American Journal of Nursing* 70:89-91, January, 1970.
The author reviews a brief but apparently effective preoperative group teaching program. The article includes a good discussion of the advantages of teaching patients in groups.

PEPLAU, HILDEGARD. "Talking with Patients." *American Journal of Nursing* 60:964-66, July, 1960.

The author discusses talking with patients as the responsible use of conversation focused on the patient and his needs rather than social chitchat that meets the nurse's needs.

RASMUSSEN, ETTA H., "Preparation for Supervising Licensed Practical Nurses." *Nursing Outlook* 10:472-75, July, 1962.
This article points out clearly the role of the professional nurse in relation to the supervision of practical nurses.

ROBINSON, GERALDINE, and FILKINS, MARILYN. "Group Teaching with Outpatients." *American Journal of Nursing* 64:110-12, November, 1964.
The constructive use of clinic waiting time is clearly shown in this article about a program for patient teaching in the outpatient department of a large urban hospital.

SCHULZ, ESTHER D. "Television Brings Drama to Clinic Patients." *American Journal of Nursing* 62:98-99, August, 1962.
This article describes teaching prenatal clinic patients by television, and emphasizes the role of the practitioner in assisting with this type of teaching.

Teaching Materials

In this chapter we will consider the value and use of teaching materials (teaching aids) appropriate to the practitioner's teaching. Broadly speaking, the materials that may be used for teaching purposes are unlimited. They may range from a picture cut from a magazine to an expensive teaching machine, from a simple poster made by the nurse to a motion picture planned and produced by hundreds of experienced craftsmen. The materials to be discussed here have been chosen on the basis of their appropriateness to the practitioner's teaching and on considerations of cost and availability. Our discussion will be divided into the following sections: (1) general considerations, (2) types of teaching materials, (3) devices for displaying teaching materials, and (4) sources of teaching materials.

GENERAL CONSIDERATIONS

Teaching materials may serve several purposes in the learning process. First, they extend the learner's sensory experience, thus adding to his perceptions and contributing new dimensions to his learning. When the nurse, in addition to talking with the learner, provides him with materials to be looked at, listened to, touched and handled, and sometimes even tasted and smelled, his concepts can be more fully developed and therefore his learning will be improved. Second, teaching aids offer an excellent opportunity to introduce variety into the nurse's teaching. The mere fact of novelty may arouse interest and curiosity and thus stimulate motivation to learn. Third, the concreteness of teaching aids may give meaning to abstractions and make complicated explanations unnecessary. "One picture is worth a thousand words" may apply to other teaching aids as well as pictures. This factor is also important in teaching people who have difficulty in understanding English.

The purpose of a teaching aid, as its name implies, is to help the teaching-learning process. This point must be kept in mind when materials are selected. Because a picture is attractive or a "gadget" has novelty does not necessarily mean that it will further an educational purpose. Teaching materials must be directly relevant to what is being taught and add some new dimension. In choosing materials, the nurse should ask: "Does the time and effort involved in presenting this aid and explaining it to the learner warrant its use? Will it add something to my teaching that I cannot provide myself?" Affirmative answers to these questions may justify its use. Using inappropriate materials takes up time that might be more profitably spent, and sometimes leads to confusion rather than clarification for the learner.

Teaching aids are intended to be an adjunct in teaching, not a replacement for the teacher. Most teaching materials do not teach in and of themselves. They require explanation, and learners need a chance to study them and to ask questions about them. Even television, which would seem to be able to teach "by itself," has been found to be more effective when a classroom teacher is on hand after the viewing to discuss the television lesson and answer the learners' questions.

Many teaching aids are representational — that is, they merely represent actual objects; for example, photographs, models, diagrams. It is important that the learners be aware of how the aids differ from reality. Photographs may be much larger or much smaller than the objects they picture; anatomical models cannot reproduce the actual color or texture of tissues and may be constructed to "come apart" in a most unlifelike way; diagrams are by definition not a true portrayal of the objects they represent. If these differences are not clearly explained, the learner may come away with some very peculiar ideas about the real characteristics of the objects represented by the aids.

The materials used in teaching can best serve the purpose of arousing the learner's interest and holding his attention if they are attractive in appearance and kept in good condition. Careful handling, protection from dust and dirt, and safe storage when not in use will prolong their usefulness. However, too much emphasis on preventing wear and tear should not be allowed to interfere with the learner's freedom to handle and examine them closely. Our impulse when someone shows us something is usually to take it in our hands in order to see it, weigh it, feel its texture; in this way we become familiar with the object by using several of our senses. This impulse should be encouraged; teaching aids should be considered to be expendable and should be replaced when necessary.

TYPES OF TEACHING MATERIALS

The choice of specific teaching aids will be determined by several factors: the topic to be presented, the particular learner or learners to be taught, the availability of the materials. We cannot, of course, mention here all the possibilities; the actual selection must be made by the nurse in each teaching situation. However, we can discuss the general types of teaching materials and make some suggestions for their use. Materials for teaching may include objects and models, various kinds of pictures and printed materials. We will also discuss how the nurse may make teaching aids, as well as the areas of programmed instruction and television as they relate to the practitioner's teaching.

Objects and Models

Both actual objects and models of objects may be used as aids in teaching. Actual objects might be such things as the instruments and equipment used in giving nursing care, such as syringes, irrigating equipment, bed linen, and so forth. Actual objects should always be used in demonstrations of nursing procedures.

Models are used when the actual object is either not available or not appropriate for use in the teaching setting. In nursing, those most often used are models of human anatomy; for example, the torso, the eye, the ear. Many of these models have removable sections that make it possible to show underlying structures and spatial relationships. Models are generally quite fragile and relatively expensive. They break easily and are not readily replaceable because of the cost; both the nurse and the learner should try to handle them carefully.

Another kind of model often used in nursing settings and probably familiar to most students of nursing is "Mrs. Chase," the adult-sized doll who substitutes for the patient, or "Baby Chase," who serves a similar purpose in pediatrics. If these models are available for teaching co-workers, they can be used to great advantage for demonstrating and practicing nursing skills. However, the learner may need to be reminded that doing a procedure for "Mrs. Chase" may be quite different from doing it for a real patient and that adjustments will have to be made in the actual situation.

Photographs

Photographs suitable for teaching purposes may be original photographic prints or illustrations from magazines, newspapers, or books. They have the advantage of being quite readily available and relatively inexpensive and are most appropriate for bulletin board displays, for posters, and for individual teaching.

Photographs and illustrations to be used in group teaching should be large enough to be seen by everyone when they are held up at the front of the room; otherwise they should be posted so that the learners can inspect them before or after the class. Passing pictures around the group diverts the learners' attention and makes it necessary to stop teaching until everyone has seen them.

It is sometimes difficult to find just the right picture when it is needed; the nurse may find it helpful to make a collection of pictures that might be useful so that they will be on hand when the appropriate occasion arises. Nurses who have some skill in using photographic equipment might plan to make their own pictures for teaching purposes, providing that permission is obtained from anyone who could be identified in the pictures. For example, photographs might be taken of adaptations of equipment to be used in caring for patients in the home or of tray setups for hospital nursing procedures. Such pictures may be enlarged without great expense.

Photographs and illustrations may be protected from wear by mounting them on a firm cardboard backing and covering them with ordinary household plastic wrap. With adequate protection and careful storage, they may be used repeatedly over a long period of time.

Slides and Filmstrips

Slides and filmstrips are still pictures designed to be projected on a screen. They are appropriate for group teaching since they can be shown to everyone at the same time and the nurse can discuss them while the class looks at them. There is no problem about the size of the picture, since projected pictures may be made larger, within limits, merely by moving the projector farther away from the screen.

Commercially made slides and filmstrips may be purchased or rented, or they can be borrowed from some sources without charge. Amateur photographers can have their negatives made into slides at a reasonable cost. The major expense involved is the cost of slide or filmstrip projectors, but if the agency has such equipment, the practitioner may be able to use these visual aids to good advantage.

Motion Pictures

Motion pictures are perhaps the best possible substitute when actual experience is not available. They mirror reality, provide variety which may be motivating, and, when sound motion pictures are used, stimulate both sight and hearing. If films and a projector for the nurse's teaching must be purchased or rented, the cost may be prohibitive. However, if a projector is available and if the agency owns appropriate films or films can be borrowed rent-free or for a small charge, the factor of expense will not be a problem.

The nurse should review the film in advance to determine whether it is appropriate both for the topic to be presented and for the learners involved. It is not wise to use a film just because someone recommended it or the title seems to indicate that the film would be suitable. First, the nurse must be sure that using the film would be the best way to meet teaching objectives. The time and effort involved in obtaining and showing a film must be justified. Second, health education films are produced for many different audiences—the general public, nursing personnel, physicians, other professional groups. A "good" film for the members of the medical profession would not necessarily be a "good" film for patients or co-workers; the film must be suited to the needs of the particular audience for which it is intended.

After deciding to use the film, the nurse will have to plan just how it is going to be used. The learners should understand why it is being shown, what they are to look for, and their responsibility for contributing to a discussion after seeing the film. This is perhaps particularly important with lay people in our "movie-conscious" society, where films are likely to be regarded as entertainment and relaxation rather than as a means of learning.

We will not discuss here the operation of a motion picture projector; if the nurse is unable to show the film, arrangements will have to be made for a projectionist. Nevertheless, there are several points about the showing of films that the nurse should know, even though someone else may operate the projector. The room to be used must be large enough to accommodate the equipment and the viewers comfortably; a convenient electrical outlet and an adequate extension cord out of the way of traffic will be needed; it must be possible to darken the room sufficiently for clear visibility; seats should be no nearer than 6 feet from the screen.

When films are to be borrowed, they should be ordered at least a month in advance and alternative dates should be specified. After use, films should be returned immediately so that other borrowers may have them in time for their scheduled showings; failure to return films promptly may mean permanent loss of borrowing privileges. Many film distributors ask that films not be rewound before returning so that they may be inspected by the distributor during the rewinding process. Borrowers are responsible for damage and loss.

Pamphlets and Posters

The practitioner will probably find that pamphlets and posters are among the most valuable teaching materials. They are available at little or no cost and often in quantity on most of the subjects the nurse will have occasion to teach. Many of them are intended for the general public and thus are well suited to most of the nurse's potential learners.

Pamphlets may be explained and given to the learner before a topic is presented in order to stimulate his interest and prepare him for the discussion, or after the teaching has been done to serve as a review and to provide additional information. Many pamphlets are so well organized that the nurse may want to use them on some occasions as a basis for a lesson.

Posters are usually designed to point up a single health principle and are intended to arouse interest rather than to give extensive information. Small-sized posters are particularly appropriate as handouts in clinics or schools and larger sizes can be used most effectively in group teaching or in bulletin board displays.

Many posters and pamphlets are printed in several languages. Obviously, such materials would be of great value in teaching people whose native language is not English.

Teacher-Made Aids

We have discussed a variety of prepared teaching materials that may be obtained from various educational or commercial sources, but we must not overlook the value of teaching aids made by the practitioner. The greatest advantage of such materials is that they may be designed to meet a specific teaching need in a particular situation. Sometimes prepared aids do not exactly meet the need or are not readily available.

Teacher-made aids do not have to be elaborate; the only requirement is that they serve their intended purpose. Nurses with even some small skill in drawing can devise posters and charts that are attractive in appearance and project a "message"; appropriate models can be constructed from a variety of materials; illustrations can be mounted on poster board with captions that will arouse interest. One of the references at the end of this chapter gives explicit instructions for beginners who want to make their own teaching aids. With some expenditure of time and imagination, the nurse can create inexpensive and appropriate teaching materials.

Programmed Instruction

Programmed instruction (or programmed learning) is a method of self-instruction that has growing significance for the nursing practitioner.

As greater numbers of programmed materials on health education are produced, the practitioner will find increasing opportunities to use them in promoting the objectives of health teaching. It is therefore important that the nurse have some understanding of what this technique is and the educational principles upon which it is based. We can do no more than touch the highlights; readers who are interested in a more detailed discussion of programmed instruction are referred to the suggested readings at the end of the chapter.

In programmed instruction, the learner studies a subject or topic by means of a teaching machine or a programmed book or pamphlet. The material to be learned is called the "program" and is made up of a series of very small segments of information arranged in a logical sequence from the very simple to the more complex. The material is presented to the learner in "frames," each one of which consists of a segment of information to be studied, followed by a question to be answered. The teaching machine or programmed book is so arranged that the learner looks at only one frame at a time; when he has written his answer in the appropriate place, he is directed to the correct answer. If his answer is incorrect, he is instructed to repeat the current frame or to go back several frames to review earlier information necessary for arriving at the correct answer. If his answer is correct, he proceeds to the next frame. He works through the entire program in this way at his own speed.

Programmed instruction is effective because it is based on learning principles. We learn by active participation: thus, the learner is required to be involved actively by reading the questions, writing in answers, and manipulating the machine or book. We are motivated to learn by the immediate reinforcement of correct responses; thus, the program is so constructed that the learner is usually able to give the correct answer and is immediately and continuously aware of his progress. Each new step in learning requires mastery of the previous step; thus, the program is made up of a logical sequence of related bits of information and the learner must answer each question correctly before he goes on to the next frame.

Television as a Teaching Aid

Television was not included in the chapter on teaching methods in this book, since this type of teaching generally requires skill and technical knowledge which involves more advanced preparation than we are discussing here. Practitioners may on occasion be asked to give a demonstration of patient care on closed-circuit television, but they would not usually carry complete responsibility for television teaching.

We have included television in this chapter as a teaching aid, however, since the practitioner may be able to plan teaching around the increasing number of television programs that present health education subjects, whether on commercial or educational television channels or on closed-circuit systems in hospitals. When it is possible to arrange for clients or co-workers to view such programs, the practitioner's function is to discuss the presentation with the learners after the viewing in order to clarify any confusion and answer questions that may be raised.

Television both as a method of teaching and as a teaching aid for the practitioner is discussed in several articles listed at the end of the chapter.

DEVICES FOR DISPLAYING TEACHING MATERIALS

Some of the teaching materials we have mentioned, such as photographs, illustrations, posters, and so forth, need some sort of device for showing them effectively. There are occasions when the nurse can merely hand them to the learner or hold them up in front of a group, but this is not always satisfactory. In this section we will discuss some of the ways of displaying teaching materials that the nurse might find helpful. Some of these devices are appropriate for use in public displays; others are suitable for individual or group teaching.

Bulletin Boards

Bulletin boards have an important place in health education, partly because they can supplement the practitioner's teaching and partly because they often reach an audience with which the nurse has little or no direct contact. When bulletin board displays are placed in the corridors or waiting rooms of hospitals, clinics, health offices, and schools, they may be seen by hundreds of people who pass by. If the display is effective, it may serve to teach many people who might not otherwise be reached.

Bulletin boards may range from expensive boards with protecting glass doors and built-in lights to those made of a wood panel covered with several layers of blotting paper, felt, or other appropriate material to allow for the insertion of thumbtacks. If a cork-covered board is used, it would be wise to remember that inserting thumbtacks over a long period of time in the same spot (for example, in the corners of the board) will eventually cause the cork to crumble and therefore it is a good idea to vary the spots where tacks are placed. If a wooden board is used, it would be advisable to put in and take out tacks with a tack hammer to avoid painful thumbs and broken fingernails. Actually, it makes little difference about the kind of board that is used—it is what is put on the board that is important.

What makes a bulletin board display effective? First is the location of the board itself. Granted that it may not always be possible to hang a board in the most advantageous location, ideally it should be placed where the lighting is good, where it can be easily seen, and where the potential audience passes by. It should be at a comfortable height for the observer; boards intended for children should be placed lower than those intended for adults.

Teaching materials should be displayed on a bulletin board that is used only for this purpose or, if a very large board is available, a section of it should be reserved just for teaching. Notices for agency employees, fire and air raid drill instructions, and similar items should be posted elsewhere so that they do not interfere with the teaching display.

In planning what to put on the board, the nurse should remember that this is one teaching aid that may instruct in the absence of the teacher. Therefore, the display must attract the observer's attention, make clear what the display is all about, and project the "message" entirely on its own merits. All this can be accomplished with careful planning.

The topic for the board must be appropriate for the potential audience and should include only one theme or idea at a time. If there are many ideas to be presented on the particular topic, a series of displays over a period of time might be planned, rather than including too much at once. Most of the people who may see the board are just passing by; the point is to catch their attention quickly and impress them with one idea. If this is accomplished, the casual passer-by may become interested enough to stop and examine future displays.

An effective display has a large, easily seen heading that states the subject of the display, some central focus for the eye, such as an attractive colored picture, and explanatory captions that are brief and to the point. Various materials, such as colored paper tape or ribbon, may be used as a border and to direct the eye in a logical path from one area of the display to another. Attention should be given to a balanced effect and even such a small detail as the use of thumbtacks of identical size and color can enhance the visual impression.

Bulletin board displays should be checked frequently after they have been set up to be sure that they are still in good condition, and after a reasonable time, the display should be changed. By storing materials that have been used, the nurse will be able to repeat an effective display or use some of the materials in a different way for future displays. It is also helpful to keep a running record of the topics used as themes and the dates during which these topics were on display.

Some estimate of the effectiveness of a teaching bulletin board may be gained from noticing whether it attracts attention, whether people are interested enough to look at it closely, and whether people ask the nurse for more information about the topic being presented. Displays that attract attention and stimulate thought and questions are serving their purpose well.

Magnetic Boards

Magnetic bulletin boards of the kind sometimes used in homes to post grocery lists or reminders to family members may be appropriate for the nurse's teaching on some occasions. These boards are made of lightweight metal, and the materials are held in place by means of small magnets instead of thumbtacks. The advantages of these boards are that they are easily portable and that the materials displayed can be quickly moved about on the board or changed; the disadvantage is that they are usually rather small, thus limiting the amount and size of the material that can be displayed. They are particularly suitable for teaching bed patients, since the nurse can easily carry them to the bedside and most patients will have little difficulty in holding and handling them. If the board is fitted with an easel back, it can be set up on the patient's bedside table instead of being held by the nurse or patient.

Flannel or Felt Boards

Flannel or felt boards are well suited for displaying materials to a group of learners during a group session. These boards may be purchased or they may be easily constructed by the nurse at little expense. The board may be made from a thin plywood panel of appropriate size, covered on one side with flannel or felt. The materials to be displayed are glued to pieces of flannel or felt that have been cut to size. When the item is placed on the board, the backing adheres to the covering of the board and the item is held in place; it is removed simply by lifting it from the board. The cloth-backed materials can be easily stored and used many times. Since no tacks or magnets are needed, items can be quickly put in place, moved, and taken off the board without interrupting the teaching that is in progress. The board may be set up on a freestanding easel, or a support may be attached to the board itself so that it can be set on a table.

Blackboards

Blackboards (or chalkboards) are another kind of device for displaying teaching materials; for example, the topic of the lesson, important concepts to be emphasized, vocabulary, and simple diagrams. In planning teaching, the nurse should first make sure that a board will be available and then decide how best to use it. Some of the material might be put on the board before the class starts, some might be written while the class is in progress. Boards and erasers must be cleaned regularly and writing or printing must be legible and large enough to be clearly visible to everyone in the group. Unless there is a specific reason for using colored chalks, it is usually best to use hard white chalk, since it is easy to see and does not streak when erased, as colored chalks and soft chalks sometimes do. Blackboards should be used sparingly and only when their use will contribute to teaching objectives; writing on a blackboard uses up valuable time and takes the nurse's attention away from the learners.

SOURCES OF TEACHING MATERIALS

There are many sources of free or inexpensive health education materials that are well adapted to the practitioner's teaching needs. These materials consist chiefly of pamphlets, posters, filmstrips, and motion pictures intended for educational purposes; in general, they are prepared by experts, kept up to date in relation to content, and presented in an attractive format. The sources of teaching materials may be classified into three categories: government-sponsored health departments; voluntary, nonprofit health organizations; and commercial sources.

There are several points of information about these materials that might be helpful to know. First, many of these organizations issue a list of their teaching materials that they will send on request. These listings generally include a brief description of the materials, the audience for whom they are intended, the cost if any, and whether the materials can be obtained in quantity. In requesting lists or materials from national organizations, your letter should be addressed to the branch office in your community or the nearest city. If there are no such offices, you may direct your inquiry to the national office. It would be wise to state in your letter that you are a nurse and would like to obtain materials for teaching purposes, particularly if you are asking for materials in quantity.

It is, of course, impossible to list here all the sources of inexpensive teaching aids that are available, but a representative listing of some of the most widely known organizations that have such materials will give the nurse a general idea of where they may be obtained. If the nurse should happen to see a particularly appropriate pamphlet or film, it would be wise to make a written note of the name and address of the organization from which the material can be obtained. It would also be helpful to compile a list of the sources of teaching materials especially relevant to the area of subject matter the practitioner teaches.

Government Health Departments

On the national level, the United States Department of Health, Education, and Welfare is the source of many excellent materials for health teaching. Inquiries for free materials should be addressed to the various special bureaus and offices of the Department. Two of these subdivisions that are especially relevant are the Children's Bureau and the United States Public Health Service. Their addresses follow:

United States Department of Health, Education, and Welfare
  Social Security Administration
  Children's Bureau
  Washington, D. C. 20203

Public Inquiries Branch, Office of Information
  U.S. Public Health Service
  Department of Health, Education, and Welfare
  Washington, D. C. 20204

Inquiries for any materials from the Department for which there is a
charge should be addressed to:
  Superintendent of Documents
  U.S. Government Printing Office
  Washington, D. C. 20204

The Office of the Superintendent of Documents also issues lists of new
publications on a wealth of subjects at frequent intervals; these lists will
be sent to anyone who requests that his name be placed on the mailing
list. There are moderate charges for the materials on these lists.

State health departments are probably among the best sources for a
variety of teaching materials. Printed materials are generally supplied
free, and films and filmstrips are loaned without charge to residents of
the state. Many of these materials are available through county and city
health department offices throughout the state; for materials that cannot
be obtained locally, address the State Health Department at the state
capital.

County and city health departments, besides serving as distribution
points for materials from the state, may also have materials particularly
suited to the educational needs of the local area; for example, pamphlets
and posters translated into the native languages of groups living in the
area or materials about certain diseases endemic in the locality.

For an excellent example of what one state health department has done
with regard to making information available about free or inexpensive
teaching materials on health and disease, see the reference listed at the
end of this chapter under the Maryland State Health Department. Other
states have similar listings of health education materials.

Voluntary Health Organizations

One of the primary purposes of our voluntary health associations and
health foundations on national, state, and local levels is education—education of both professional personnel and the general public. Some of
these organizations have general materials on promoting health and preventing illness; others, which are devoted to education and research

on particular diseases have very specialized materials (heart disease, diabetes, and so forth). Listed below is a small sampling of these organizations. The addresses given are for the national headquarters, but local chapters or branch offices should be contacted whenever possible. The practitioner should not find it difficult to locate information about health organizations not included here.

American Association for Health, Physical Education, and Recreation
    1201 16th Street N.W., Washington, D. C. 20036
American Cancer Society
    219 East 42nd Street, New York, New York 10017
American Dental Association
    211 East Chicago Avenue, Chicago, Illinois 60611
American Diabetes Association
    18 East 48th Street, New York, New York 10017
American Dietetic Association
    620 North Michigan Avenue, Chicago, Illinois 60611
American Heart Association
    44 East 23rd Street, New York, New York 10010
American Hospital Association
    840 North Lake Shore Drive, Chicago, Illinois 60611
American Medical Association
    535 North Dearborn Street, Chicago, Illinois 60610
American Nurses' Association
    10 Columbus Circle, New York, New York 10019
American Public Health Association
    1015 18th Street, N.W., Washington, D. C. 20036
American Red Cross
    Contact local office only
Child Study Association of America
    9 East 89th Street, New York, New York 10028
Health Education Service
    P.O. Box 7283 Capitol Station, Albany, New York 12201
Mental Health Materials Center
    419 Park Avenue South, New York, New York 10016
National Association for Mental Health
    10 Columbus Circle, New York, New York 10019
National Education Association
    1201 16th Street N.W., Washington, D. C. 20036
The National Foundation, Division of Scientific and Health Information
    800 2nd Avenue, New York, New York 10017
National Health Council
    1740 Broadway, New York, New York 10019

National League for Nursing
    10 Columbus Circle, New York, New York 10019
National Safety Council
    425 North Michigan Avenue, Chicago, Illinois 60611
National Tuberculosis and Respiratory Disease Association
    Contact local office only

Commercial Sources

There are many business enterprises that distribute teaching materials
about health and illness. Although they are profit-making organizations,
some of them have special departments designated to prepare and distribute health education materials, usually without charge. These firms
are all concerned either directly or indirectly with health or illness: in-
surance, pharmaceuticals, medical and hospital supplies, food, dairy products, personal hygiene, and so forth. The addresses of these firms may
sometimes be found in their advertisements in professional or lay magazines or in the literature that is packed with their products. Some of these
businesses have branch offices in major cities and their addresses may be
found in local telephone directories.

A few words of warning are necessary about using teaching materials
that advertise commercial products. It sometimes happens, although it
is not always the case, that the information is slanted in favor of the
product the company is selling and there is consequently a bias expressed.
Another point of importance is that the nurse should clear with someone in authority in the agency as to whether materials containing adver-
tising may be used for the general public, lest the learner conclude that
the agency is officially recommending the product.

SUMMARY

The teaching materials and aids discussed in this chapter are those
that the practitioner might reasonably use in teaching in nursing settings.
Nurses should not expect to use every aid we have mentioned; on the
other hand, they should not limit themselves only to those we have discussed. With experience, good judgment, and a little imagination, the
practitioner will be able to recognize materials that would be appropriate and that would make teaching and learning more effective.

REFERENCES

BORGERS, HANNAH M. "Televising Health Lessons in School." *American Journal
    of Nursing* 63:96-98, June, 1963.
    The author, a school nurse, describes the planning and televising of a series
    of health lessons for school children and evaluates the outcomes.

Horn, George F. *Bulletin Boards*. New York: Reinhold Publishing Corporation, 1962.
This small book presents many ingenious and inexpensive ideas for teacher-made bulletin board displays. The value of the book is enhanced by very effective and amusing illustrations.

Kinsella, Cynthia. "Educational Television for a Hospital System." *American Journal of Nursing* 64:72-76, January, 1964.
This article discusses the development and production of a television teaching program as an effective tool for in-service education in a large municipal hospital system.

Linden, Kathryn. "The Multimedia Approach to Teaching Nursing." *Nursing Outlook* 17:36-40, May, 1969.
This article was written for teachers of students of nursing, but it will have value to the practitioner in relation to patient teaching as an excellent overview of a variety of audiovisual materials.

Lysaught, Jerome P., and Williams, Clarence M. *A Guide to Programmed Instruction*. New York: John Wiley & Sons, Inc., 1963.
The authors present the history and theoretical basis of programmed instruction and clearly describe how programs are developed, tested, and evaluated.

Maryland State Department of Health, *A Guide Book Describing Pamphlets, Posters, Films on Health and Disease*, 2d ed. Baltimore: The Department, 1964.
This guide contains over 100 pages of detailed information about free or inexpensive teaching materials and includes an extensive list of sources.

Mechner, Francis. "Learning by Doing Through Programmed Instruction." *American Journal of Nursing* 65:98-104, May, 1965.
This article provides an introduction to the theoretical basis of programmed instruction, its value in teaching, and how programs are constructed. Examples of program frames are given.

Melody, Mary M., and Carrington, Lucy G. "Poster Explosion." *American Journal of Nursing* 62:92-93, August, 1962.
This article about a spontaneous poster campaign to which nursing staff, patients, and families contributed suggests possibilities for stimulating bulletin board displays for patient teaching.

Minor, Ed. *Simplified Techniques for Preparing Visual Instructional Materials*. New York: McGraw-Hill Book Company, 1962.
This book explains and illustrates how to prepare teaching materials for use. A glossary of terms and a list of sources of the materials needed are included.

Rich, Lois E. "Volunteers Plan a School Health Exhibit." *Nursing Outlook* 13:35-38, February, 1965.
This article discusses the bulletin board as a tool for a school health project and includes specific instructions and illustrations of the materials used in the displays.

Chapter ———— **8**

Planning for Teaching

In the previous chapters of this book we have discussed many concepts essential for the successful performance of the nurse's teaching function. Now we will consider how the practitioner may apply these concepts to broad overall planning for teaching and to the development of teaching guides for specific lessons.

The practitioner's teaching efforts will be more effective if an overall plan for the total teaching program in a particular setting is developed. Sporadic and uncoordinated teaching may meet a particular learner's immediate need and indicate the nurse's good intentions, but fragmented teaching activities are not likely to accomplish the broad objectives of the practitioner's teaching function. The recommendations made in this chapter are based on the fundamental premise of this book: *effective teaching is planned teaching.* Regardless of whether the teaching is done in a classroom setting using a written guide or whether it is conducted informally at the bedside without any kind of written notes, *teaching which is planned for and included in the overall program is more effective teaching.*

Planning for teaching will be discussed under the following headings: (1) planning the overall teaching program, (2) preparing teaching guides, and (3) an example of a teaching guide.

PLANNING THE OVERALL TEACHING PROGRAM

The planning of the overall teaching program is as much a part of the nurse's teaching function as is actual teaching. In hospitals and public health agencies where several practitioners work together, this planning might well be a cooperative effort by all the practitioners concerned, perhaps assisted by the head nurse or the public health supervisor; in medical offices, schools, and industry, where nurses work alone, each nurse will have to assume this responsibility, although physicians, teachers, or industrial supervisors may be asked for suggestions for the program. General planning includes predicting probable learning needs and developing a written program outline.

Predicting Probable Learning Needs

The first essential in general planning is determining the probable health education needs of the learners. These needs will, of course, vary from learner to learner, but it is possible to predict what most clients and co-workers in a particular setting will probably need to be taught. A list of relevant topics can be developed from material from a variety of sources: the practitioner's nursing knowledge and experience, what physicians may want their patients to be taught, what is expected of co-workers in giving nursing care. Other topics may be suggested by questions frequently asked by patients, parents, or co-workers, and through consultation with professional people concerned with health care.

The list might include topics about promoting health and preventing disease, as outlined in Chapter 5, as well as topics directly related to the particular health problems usually treated in this service or agency. This approach to general planning will not only indicate the extent of the teaching to be done, but may also reveal something about teaching priorities; it may become clear which topics are essential and which ones might be delayed or even omitted if the time or opportunity for teaching is limited.

As an example, let us look at a partial list of topics as it might be developed by an individual nurse or a group of nurses on a general surgical ward in a hospital. The topics for patients and families are kept separate from those proposed for co-workers.

I. Topics for patients and/or families
   A. Topics relevant for all clients
      1. Orientation to the hospital
      2. Promotion of health and prevention of illness
      3. . . .
   B. Topics relevant for all surgical patients
      1. Orientation to surgery, surgical procedures, etc.
      2. Need for postoperative positioning, turning, etc.
      3. . . .
   C. Topics relevant for patients with chest surgery
      1. Coughing and breathing exercises

       2. Explanation of suctioning, oxygen apparatus, etc.
       3. . . .
   D. Topics relevant for patients with abdominal surgery
       1. . . .
   E. Topics relevant for other surgical patients, etc.
II. Topics for co-workers
   A. Topics relevant for all co-workers
       1. Orientation to the hospital
       2. Promotion of health and prevention of illness
       3. General supportive nursing care
       4. . . .
   B. Topics relevant for co-workers on all surgical wards
       1. Preoperative and postoperative nursing care
       2. Assisting with surgical dressings
       3. . . .
   C. Topics relevant for co-workers on this unit
       1. Special nursing care in chest surgery
       2. Special nursing care in abdominal surgery
       3. . . .

Thus, the topical outline is developed. If it is possible for all the practitioners on the service to plan teaching together, not only will there be the advantage of more sources of ideas, but also much duplication of effort may be avoided. For example, topics under A and B for both clients and co-workers could be included in the teaching for all the wards in the service; topics under C, D, and E, which relate to specialties, could be planned by the nurse or nurses in those particular units.

Developing a Written Program Outline

The proposed list of topics serves as a basis for developing a written outline of the total teaching program. With this list as a starting point, overall objectives may be formulated, as discussed in Chapter 3, to insure that the program will be consistent with the practitioner's teaching goals. The outline of topics may be expanded to include definite suggestions for the details of subject matter of each topic, appropriate methods of teaching, as discussed in Chapter 6, and suitable teaching materials, as suggested in Chapter 7. Arrangements might be made at this time for a place to file program plans, teaching guides, and teaching materials so that they will be in order and easily accessible to anyone concerned with the teaching program.

As in any kind of program planning, this preliminary work is subject to additions and revisions: experience with the program may reveal other topics; changes in medical or nursing treatments or the use of new apparatus may make additional teaching necessary; effective teaching efforts may stimulate the learners' interest in other topics. Such modifications should be expected and encouraged. In general, a teaching program that is considered to be complete and "all taken care of" is likely to be a program that is inflexible and soon outdated.

PREPARING TEACHING GUIDES

A teaching guide is a written outline of the salient points of a specific lesson. Its first and most important purpose is to organize the lesson by clarifying teaching objectives, stating the methods and materials to be used, giving details of the subject matter to be discussed, and describing the activities planned both for the teacher and for the learners. The guide may also sometimes serve as a reference for the teacher while teaching is in progress.

There are many ways of setting up teaching guides; the form presented here is a simple plan that includes the essentials for planning and conducting teaching in nursing settings. An outline of the suggested guide follows; each item will be discussed, after which an example of the planning and writing of a specific teaching guide will be presented. Although the sections of the guide are discussed here in sequence, in actually planning a lesson certain areas must be developed concurrently; for example, the overall topic, the objectives, and the content to be taught are so interdependent that decisions on any one of these areas may require changes in the other two. Thus, the plan must be developed as a whole, with continual reference back and forth, so that the final guide is consistent throughout.

Agency or Service

The nursing setting in which the guide is to be used is stated to identify the teaching program for which the guide has been prepared. In some cases the particular ward, clinic, or local health office within the agency should also be specified.

Topic

The statement of the overall topic of the lesson defines and limits the scope of the content and therefore should be carefully worded. It should be stated briefly but with enough detail to show clearly what the content will be. For example, "Diabetes" as a title for a patient teaching guide is certainly brief, but gives no indication of what aspects of diabetes are to be covered; on the other hand, "The Importance of Diet in Diabetes" briefly specifies the nature of the lesson.

OUTLINE FOR TEACHING GUIDE

Agency or Service:
Topic:
Learners:
Teacher's Objectives:
Method(s) of Teaching:
Materials:

Subject Matter	Teacher and Learner Activities
1.	
A.	
B.	
C. etc.	
2.	
A.	
B.	
C. etc.	
3.	
A. etc.	
Summary:	
1. etc.	

References:

Prepared by: Date:

Learners

The learners for whom the guide has been planned should be indicated; for example, children in the third grade, prenatal clinic patients, nursing assistants on the orthopedic service, home health aides, and so forth.

Teacher's Objectives

The formulation of objectives has been discussed elsewhere. It is important to remember that in a brief lesson, objectives must be limited in scope and number; broad, general objectives belong in the total teaching program, not in specific lessons. No objectives should be included in the guide that cannot reasonably be accomplished during the lesson.

Method(s) of Teaching

The guide should show whether discussion, demonstration, or a combination of the two is to be used and whether the lesson has been planned for individual or group teaching.

Materials

Teaching materials for the lesson are enumerated and the sources where they may be obtained are indicated. Pamphlets and films are listed by title; equipment for demonstrations is itemized. The practitioner's copies of pictures, diagrams, and so forth may be attached to the guide; otherwise the place where they are filed should be stated. Any accessory equipment needed, such as blackboard and chalk, flannel board, projector, and screen, should be included. The nurse should be able to locate and assemble easily all the materials to be used by referring to this section of the guide.

Subject Matter

Subject matter is arranged in the left column in outline form, using phrases and key words rather than complete sentences. If the subject matter is written out in complete sentences, it will be necessary to pause to read every sentence silently and then say it aloud, or else just read the entire lesson to the class. Many of us have probably had the misfortune to have a teacher who read his notes; one cannot help but think, "Why doesn't he just give us mimeographed copies and let us go home and read it for ourselves in comfort?" Another point is worth mentioning—it is easier to find your place on the plan in skeleton outline form than in the solid text of sentences and paragraphs. When you become more experienced and depend very little on the guide, this point will not matter as much; when you are just beginning to do structured teaching, it will be very important for you to be able to find your place quickly.

The outline will include an introduction, the subject matter to be taught, and a summary of the major points in the lesson. The steps of a simple demonstration may be outlined after the introduction; when complex nursing care is to be demonstrated, a copy of the procedure as it appears in the agency procedure manual may be inserted in the plan.

Teacher and Learner Activities

In the column on the right, the activities planned for the teacher and learners are listed directly opposite the subject matter to which they refer; thus, as the lesson progresses, the nurse will be reminded of the activity at the point where it is to be carried out. These activities may include the questions the nurse has planned in advance to stimulate discussion and to bring out important points, distributing pamphlets, outlining points on the blackboard, putting illustrations on the flannel board, asking learners to discuss their experience, showing and explaining equipment, asking someone to summarize. Thus, this column contains instructions to the nurse for class activities. A large part of class time is devoted to the nurse's talking and directing discussion and the learners' answering and asking questions; these particular activities are taken for granted and are therefore not written in the activity column. Underlining planned questions or comments in this column will serve to draw attention to them during the lesson.

Summary of the Lesson

Good teaching includes a summary of the major points of the lesson. The summary may be given by the nurse or by one or several learners. The points to be reviewed are usually listed to avoid omissions. It is suggested that the last entry in the activity column, placed after the summary, might be, "Are there any questions?" to be sure that everyone has an opportunity to clarify any points that might be confusing.

References

If particular books or articles have been used extensively in preparing the lesson, acknowledgment is made in the references. In addition, if the nurse has found other reference materials that the learners or other teaching practitioners might find of interest, these may also be included, even though the nurse has not used them directly in the lesson. Correct bibliographic form should be used; one acceptable format is used in the references in this book.

Practitioner's Name; Date of Plan

The name of the nurse (or nurses) who developed the guide should be noted, as well as the month and year when the plan was completed. This information will be helpful when plans are made to review teaching guides for possible revision.

AN EXAMPLE OF A TEACHING GUIDE

In this section we will follow the steps in preparing a teaching guide. The reader is reminded that, although this plan is of course limited to one setting, one group of learners, and one topic, the application of teaching and learning principles would be relevant to any teaching guide.

Let us assume that the nursing staff of a pediatric outpatient clinic has become concerned over the number of small children brought to the clinic with serious injuries sustained in their homes; the most prevalent injuries have been poisoning, burns, and injuries from falls. The staff has decided to arrange a series of classes on home accident prevention for mothers in the neighborhood, many of whom speak only Spanish. Classes will be arranged for the hour before clinic sessions begin and announcements in English and Spanish will be posted in both adult and pediatric clinics, stating what the classes will be about, when they will meet, and that the mothers may leave their children in the clinic playroom during classes. The staff has suggested several topics for group discussion; the first will be concerned with accidental poisoning, and a staff nurse has agreed to give this class. We are interested in both the preliminary planning for this lesson and the guide the nurse develops.

General knowledge about the prospective learners is essential in determining how to present this material. The mothers are from a low-income group; few have had more than grade school education, and many are recent arrivals from Puerto Rico and Cuba who speak almost no English. In consequence, simple English must be used and the members of the group who are bilingual will be asked to interpret for those whose English is limited. The discussion of poisons will be limited to the products these particular women would be likely to use in their homes.

Teaching materials for this lesson will include pictures of poisonous products rather than the actual items. There are several very good reasons for this. First is the effort and expense of buying these products and arranging for their safe storage until the next time this class is conducted. Second is the convenience of having pictures that can be easily filed in a small space. Third, but certainly most important, is the fact that the nurse is trying to teach these mothers to keep poisonous household products stored in safe places—having poisons placed out on a table in plain view and easily accessible would completely negate the main point of the lesson.

With the help of various members of the pediatric clinic staff, the following materials have been prepared for this lesson and will be presented during the lesson in this order:

1. Flannel-backed materials
   a. Caption—POISON

    b. Pictures—insecticide, laundry bleach, home permanent wave kit, children's aspirin, nonprescription sleeping pills, household cleaning agents

2. Poster
    a. Caption—HANDLE WITH CARE
    b. Pictures—a dozen labels from common household products showing clearly the word "poison" and on some, the skull and crossbones symbol
    c. Printed phrases—"For external use only," "Keep away from children," "Antidote," "Call physician," "Call doctor," "Caution"

3. Flannel-backed materials
    a. Caption—DANGER!
    b. Pictures—simple line drawing showing a container marked "poison" standing unattended on a kitchen table, an under-the-sink closet with the door open showing a bottle marked "bleach," and a bathroom wall cabinet with open door showing toilet articles and medicine bottles marked "poison" on the same shelf.

It will be noted how often the word "poison" appears in the illustrative materials and that the skull and crossbones symbol will be used in the poster. It is hoped that during this session, all the learners will become familiar with the kinds of poisonous materials they may have in their homes and that the members of the group who cannot read English will hereafter recognize the word "poison" and the skull and crossbones symbol and their significance.

The completed teaching guide is presented on the following pages. Details of the guide are shown for several headings; other headings are merely listed but not developed further. It is suggested that the reader study the guide carefully, noting the applications of teaching and learning principles, and thinking of other ways to present this lesson effectively.

SUMMARY

The effectiveness of the practitioner's teaching will, of course, depend primarily on the nurse's basic knowledge of the subject being taught; it will also depend on the quality of the overall advance planning, the care with which plans for individual lessons or teaching incidents are prepared and presented, and painstaking evaluation. We have tried in this chapter to show how the nurse finally applies the principles we have been emphasizing throughout the book. Only one teaching guide has been presented, but it is hoped that the nurse will be able to prepare other lessons with this plan as a guide.

Agency: X Hospital Outpatient Department, Pediatric Clinic
Topic: Prevention of Accidental Poisoning of Children in the Home
Learners: Mothers attending outpatient department clinics
Objectives:
1. To help mothers recognize potential poisoning hazards in the home
2. To help mothers plan how to eliminate or minimize these hazards
Method: Group discussion
Materials: Flannel board and easel (supply closet, supervisor's office)
Flannel-backed materials (clinic teaching file under HOME SAFETY)
POISON; DANGER!
Poster (supply closet, pediatric clinic office)
HANDLE WITH CARE

Subject Matter	Teacher and Learner Activities
1. Introduction A. 32 children poisoned last year in this neighborhood B. We can do something about it C. This is the purpose of this class	Welcome mothers and introduce yourself. Seat "interpreters" where needed. Ask interpreters to translate *poisoned*.
2. Common household poisons	Put up caption POISON. Do you have any poisons in your home? Put up illustrations mentioned by class; add those not mentioned. Now let's talk more about these poisons.

A. Products used to kill pests
  1. For ants, roaches, mice, etc.
  2. Spays, powders, pastes
B. Laundry and cleaning supplies
  1. Germ killers (disinfectants)
  2. Bleach, ammonia, lye, etc.
	Can you think of any others?
	Ask interpreters if Spanish-speaking mothers have suggestions.

Subject Matter	Teacher and Learner Activities

C. Cosmetics
  1. Waving solution, hair coloring
  2. Deodorants, polish remover
D. Paints and painting supplies
  1. Paints containing lead
  2. Turpentine, thinner, etc.
E. Medicines
  1. etc.
	Do any of you give yourselves or your children <u>permanents at home?</u>
	
	How can your child get sick from the paint on his <u>toys or his crib?</u>

3. Recognizing poisons A. "Poison"; "antidote" B. "For external use only" C. "Keep away from children" D. etc.	How can we tell that something is a poison? Put poster HANDLE WITH CARE on easel and discuss labels and phrases in detail; then set poster aside.
4. Preventing poisoning accidents A. etc.	Where should we store poisons? Put up caption DANGER! Ask for ideas; put up illustrations.
5. If you think your child is poisoned A. etc.	What do you think you should do if you think <u>your child is poisoned?</u>
Summary: A. Know what poisons you have at home. B. Store poisons safely. C. Never leave small children alone. D. Know what to do if an accident happens.	Nurse summarizes. <u>Are there any questions?</u>

Reference: American National Red Cross, *First Aid Textbook*, rev. ed., Garden City, N. Y.: Doubleday & Company, Inc., 1966.

Prepared by: Mary Rogers   Date: January, 19____.

REFERENCES

ABBOTT, NANCY C., et al. "Dress Rehearsal for the Hospital." *American Journal of Nursing* 70:2360-62, November, 1970.
This delightfully illustrated article gives the details of planning and carrying out a class for kindergarten children about going to the hospital.

ELLIOTT, HAL. "A Traction Workshop for Orderlies." *Nursing Outlook* 18:47, March, 1970.
This brief article explains clearly the steps followed in planning and evaluating a workshop for orderlies.

HAFERJORN, VIRGINIA. "Assessing Individual Needs as a Basis for Patient Teaching." *Nursing Clinics of North America* 6:199-209, March, 1971.
This is an excellent, detailed article on assessing patient's needs before teaching is planned. The author outlines a four-point approach to planning patient teaching and proceeds to develop these points.

HAHN, ANNE, and DOLAN, NANCY. "After Coronary Care—Then What?" *American Journal of Nursing* 70:2350-52, November, 1970.
This article discusses the what, who, and when of teaching the patient who has had a myocardial infarction. Planning with the family is included. The article ends with a concise summary of what the nurses learned during this study.

HALLBURG, JEANNE C. "Teaching Patients Self-Care." *Nursing Clinics of North America* 5:223-32, June, 1970.
This article is concerned with teaching outpatients in a hospital clinic, planning both for and with the patient. The article concludes with a most interesting section, "An Experiment: Planning with Patients."

JARVIS, MARILYN A., PULLEN, MARY, and DOWNIN, JANE. "Health Larnin' in Appalachia." *American Journal of Nursing* 67:2345-47, November, 1967.
This is a fascinating article on the development of plans for health teaching in the mountains of West Virginia. Families who knew nearly nothing about health were motivated to learn by the way the nurses who taught them got them involved in planning.

REDMAN, BARBARA K. *The Process of Patient Teaching in Nursing.* St. Louis: C. V. Mosby, 1968.
Certain sections of this book have been mentioned in other chapter references. Anyone who is planning overall patient teaching and working out specific teaching guides will find much helpful material throughout this book.

SCHWEER, JEAN E. *Creative Teaching in Clinical Nursing.* St. Louis: C. V. Mosby, 1968.
Although this book has been written for teachers in basic programs for nursing, it has much to offer the practitioner who is planning teaching, especially in the sections dealing with methods and materials (pp. 144-239) and the evaluation of teaching and learning experiences in the clinical setting (pp. 240-269).

SHEA, KATHLEEN, and others. "Teaching a Patient to Live with Adrenal Insufficiency." *American Journal of Nursing* 65:80-85, December, 1965.
This article contains a guide for patient teaching. The reader's attention is called to the sections on the teaching program, patients' questions, and evaluation.

VARVARO, FILOMENA FANELLI. "Teaching the Patient About Open Heart Surgery." *American Journal of Nursing* 65:111-15, October, 1965.
This article discusses how a nursing instructor and her students developed a plan for teaching preoperative open-heart surgery patients and evaluated the results of the teaching.

WONNELL, EDITH B. "The Education of the Expectant Father for Childbirth." *Nursing Clinics of North America* 6:591-603, December, 1971.
This is an interesting article in terms of its content, but it would also be of value in terms of planning and good organization of the materials used. The instruction sheets for fathers for helping their wives during labor are models of clarity and simplicity.

Evaluating Teaching
and Learning

This chapter is devoted to one of the most important aspects of teaching—evaluation. Evaluation of the practitioner's teaching includes an assessment of the nurse's performance as a teacher and the performance of the client or the co-worker as a learner. Since teaching is the avenue by which objectives are realized and learning is the end product, both teaching and learning must be considered in order to produce a meaningful evaluation. We will discuss some general considerations and then look at evaluating the learning of our clients and co-workers, the appraisal of the nursing care given by co-workers, and the evaluation of the teacher and the teaching.

GENERAL CONSIDERATIONS

Evaluation is a process of appraisal, of estimating the worth or value of something. "Something" may be a person, an object, an activity, a belief. In the teaching-learning situation, evaluation is the process by which the teacher attempts to arrive at a judgment of the effectiveness of the teaching and the learning that has taken place. This process requires careful attention and study, and must be systematic and continuing. Evaluation is perhaps one of the most difficult and at the same time one of the most important parts of teaching.

Evaluation occurs every day of our lives. It is taking place when we say (or think), "I really made a mess out of that job," or "That was a good television show," or "I think that new patient is very nice." Or we make this kind of evaluative remark: "She criticized me unfairly; I don't think *her* technique is so special, either!" or "He (or she) is the most wonderful person in the world!" All of these remarks are evaluative—

that is, they express a judgment about the worth of something, but, in general, they are personal opinions that may not be supported by actual evidence, and are therefore not necessarily valid.

At this point it might be worthwhile to look at our own attitudes about evaluation, since many of us have mixed feelings about the subject. In the light of some of our past experiences, we are likely to equate evaluation with criticism and fault-finding. With respect to the word *criticism,* it is interesting that the usual connotation of the word is negative, when actually criticism is as much concerned with the positive as with the negative. As to "faultfinding," it is true that discovering weaknesses is one aspect of the process, but it is by no means the sole or primary purpose of evaluation. Evaluation should be viewed, by both the evaluator and the person being evaluated, as a process intended to point out what is good as well as what needs to be corrected, to stimulate the desire for improvement and to encourage further effort. If the nurse is able to accept this viewpoint and convey it to the people being evaluated, the process will be more likely to serve its ultimate purpose—to improve the practitioner's teaching and, consequently, the client's learning.

OBJECTIVITY AND SUBJECTIVITY

A major characteristic of worthwhile evaluation is objectivity. Webster defines the adjective *objective* as: "Exhibiting or characterized by emphasis upon, or the tendency to view events, phenomena, ideas, etc., as external and apart from self-consciousness; not subjective; hence, detached; impersonal; unprejudiced." The same source defines *subjective* as: "Exhibiting or affected by personal bias, emotional background, etc." The evaluator must try to be as objective as possible, if the resulting appraisal is to be sound.

The value of subjectivity is not being negated here. Subjectivity must be minimized as far as possible in evaluation, because letting personal feelings govern our judgment often blinds us to the real situation. However, there are many times in life when subjectivity is not only important but necessary—in personal relationships, in working in the creative arts such as painting, writing, music and the dance, and in enjoying those arts. These are just a few examples; it is clear that they may all require emotional involvement—subjectivity.

It is very easy, of course, to say, "Be objective," and sometimes very hard to do. Our appraisals are not objective when our emotions are out of control, often because of something entirely outside of the evaluation setting: we are not feeling well, something has gone wrong at home, we have just been evaluated ourselves and the results are not what we would have liked to hear. We all recognize such a situation when we hear remarks like: "I hope she had a good night's sleep last night," or "He must have eaten something that disagreed with him," or "She must have gotten up on the wrong side of the bed."

Psychologists and educators use the phrase *halo effect* to describe a subjective reaction that is carried over to a new situation regardless of the evidence in the new situation. The word *halo* implies "angelic" or "able to do no wrong." When we have formed a very positive reaction to a person (possibly based on sound evidence), we tend to associate him with a positive aura in other settings. Thus when this person does a poor piece of work we think, "Well, he just had an off day today; that's not his usual performance." On the other hand, if we have had reason to form a negative opinion of someone, we are more likely to look closely for things to find fault about, and perhaps even ignore the fact that he has done a very good job. This worker "can't win" when we are his evaluators.

Stereotypes, which we discussed in Chapter 3, can be just as detrimental to fair evaluation as the halo effect. If we have had just one or two opportunities to observe, for example, a Japanese worker, and each time he did a superior piece of work, we may expect the same caliber of work from the next Japanese worker we observe. If he does not measure up to our stereotype of Japanese workers, we may either make excuses for him or we may decide that our previous impression of Japanese workers was wrong and therefore change it.

It is important to be aware that halo effects and stereotypes may be unconscious and therefore unknown to us. If this is the case, they can be dislodged only by our being aware that they may exist and examining our evaluative judgments very carefully for evidence of their presence. Once we recognize any of these mechanisms, the battle is half over. On the conscious level we can keep reminding ourselves that Mr. A. has a halo or Miss B. is Japanese; the halo or stereotype may still be our first involuntary response, but if we recognize it, we will have a chance to prevent its influencing our evaluations.

Here is another example of subjectivity in evaluation: if you persist in doing something I approve of, you are resolute and tenacious; if I do not approve of it, you are stubborn and obstinate. Notice how the particular words I use color my appraisal—*resolute* is "good," *stubborn* is "bad."

The pinning of "good" and "bad" labels on people constitutes making moral judgments. Moral means conforming to a standard of what is right and good. The question, of course, is, "right and good according to whose standards?" As nurses we are entitled (and expected) to make judgments about nursing care, about how patients are responding to medical therapy, about what they need to be taught about their health; as nurses, it is *not* our concern to decide whether we think an individual lives an up-right life, about whether he conforms to *our* standards of what is right. If we accept the person as he is, we will be better able to help him; if he feels that acceptance through our behavior toward him, he will be better able to take our help. It is essential to remember that our responsibility for evaluation includes only how well our client or co-worker performs in the light of what we tried to teach him. Therefore, we appraise the *activity*, not the *person*.

During the process of evaluation, perhaps the best way to try to maintain objectivity is to check on ourselves frequently. Are we judging *today's* performance? Are we keeping our personal feeling out of it? Is it very important to us to be liked and is that entering into the way we evaluate? Are we using the same standards of appraisal for everyone, regardless of previous performance? Do we recognize that everyone who does evaluating is subject at one time or another to the influence of halos or stereotypes? If we earnestly try to eliminate subjectivity in our evaluating, we will certainly approach the objectivity that is important in sound appraisals.

EVALUATION AND OBJECTIVES

The starting point in any evaluation is a careful review of objectives. In Chapter 3 we discussed three reasons for setting up objectives; namely, to make clear what is to be accomplished in the teaching, to give direction for planning the teaching, and to serve as the key to the evaluation of teaching and learning. It is this last purpose that has particular relevance here.

Objectives are set up to state what goals we hope to reach in our teaching, whether in a single brief lesson or in a total teaching program. Evaluation is carried out to show us whether or not we (and our learners) actually did reach those goals. In retrospect, evaluation may also show us whether the objectives we have set up are clearly stated and realistic. If any of them are found to be ambiguous or unrealistic, they can be clarified or, in some cases, discarded, and new objectives set up. Clearly, evaluation and objectives are closely related to each other in teaching and learning.

EVALUATING THE LEARNING OF CLIENTS AND CO-WORKERS

How can we judge whether our client or co-worker has learned what we have tried to teach him? Since learning is an intellectual process that requires time and further experience to be thoroughly assimilated, it is not always possible to determine directly and immediately how well the learner has grasped what we have taught. However, there are some indications of successful learning that the practitioner may observe, both during and after the teaching, upon which judgments can be made. Can the learner rephrase in his own words the concepts that have been presented? Is he able to apply what we have taught him in actual situations? After sufficient practice, can he perform what he has seen demonstrated? Does he ask questions that indicate a grasp of the material that was taught?

Questions about our planning for teaching may also be helpful in evaluating learning. Were our objectives clearly formulated and sufficiently limited so that it was possible to achieve them? Did we estimate accurately the learning needs of the client or co-worker, his intellectual ability, his motivation to learn? Did we constantly apply the principles of learning as we taught? Was our communication effective and was there evidence of good teacher-learner rapport?

These questions can be answered only if the practitioner keeps in mind the importance of evaluation at all stages of the teaching process— in planning, in actual teaching, and in follow-up. It is probable that the inexperienced teacher will find this to be most difficult during the stage of actual teaching because of the involvement with content and techniques. However, as skill improves and the nurse feels more at ease with the technical aspects of teaching, it will be possible to develop the habit of making mental notes about what is happening during a teaching session for later consideration. Each session should be analyzed as soon as possible. If the evaluation must be delayed, brief written notes should be made so that points to be considered will not be forgotten in the meantime.

The teacher in the school setting may make use of a variety of techniques and tools to evaluate learning; for example, written assignments, oral and written quizzes, formal examinations, and written progress records of student achievement. In most nursing situations, however, such direct techniques are not appropriate and the practitioner will generally have to depend on less formal, less direct methods of evaluation.

EVALUATING THE CO-WORKER'S NURSING CARE

In the chapter on methods of teaching, we discussed teaching the co-worker through supervising and evaluating the nursing care given to patients. The areas included were supervision as a cooperative relationship, knowledge about the work and the worker, and skillful observation. A fourth point, constructive evaluation, was mentioned and will be discussed here.

After the practitioner has made observations, there should be a discussion with the worker as soon as possible about what has been observed. By constructive evaluation we mean assessment of what is good about the worker's performance as well as what needs improvement. Too often evaluations focus on weak points and neglect strengths. All of us need the encouragement of knowing that our good points are recognized; it makes it easier to face the problem of improving our weaknesses.

Constructive evaluation also implies that specific suggestions for improvement are made. It is not very helpful merely to tell someone his work is unsatisfactory; he must know in what way it is unsatisfactory and what he can do to improve. It is at this point that the teaching aspect of supervision becomes paramount. The nurse by this time will have specific knowledge about the worker's educational and experience background, a picture of his strengths and weaknesses, and a clear idea of how his performance measures up to the standards of nursing care expected in this particular nursing unit. On the basis of this information, the nurse will be able to plan the evaluation conference and determine what the worker still needs to learn and the best way of teaching him.

We have mentioned the importance of two-way communication between the practitioner and the worker. The evaluation conference should be a two-way process. Instead of conducting the session as though it were a lecture by the nurse, a good beginning is to ask the worker how he thinks he is progressing or what his feelings are about the day's assignment. This may serve several constructive purposes: mutual communication can be established immediately and may continue throughout the conference, and the worker will have the opportunity to express feelings which might otherwise block his participation in the evaluation. Another result may be that the worker will be encouraged to evaluate himself. The person who is encouraged to evaluate himself is more likely to develop the habit of self-evaluation and will gradually need less direction from someone else in improving his performance. At the same time the nurse will be able to see what insights the learner has already developed and what further help he may need.

When the nurse discusses what has been observed, it is a good practice to begin with the worker's strong points and the satisfactory aspects of his work, partly because this will encourage him and partly because these points are sometimes not mentioned if the discussion begins with areas that need to be improved. When weaknesses are discussed, the worker should share in the discussion and be encouraged to attempt to decide why parts of his work are unsatisfactory and how he might improve. The more the worker is able to criticize his own work, the more the habit of self-evaluation will be strengthened. Concrete suggestions should be made as part of the conference; for example, perhaps the worker needs more practice in using certain equipment that he has had trouble in handling, or maybe he could improve his skill in observing patients' symptoms by trying to assess each patient's condition and then discussing his observations with the nurse. Some sort of brief but pertinent notes should be kept about what suggestions and plans have been made as a point of reference for future conferences.

The nurse should pay attention to how the worker reacts to the suggestions made, both during the conference and subsequently in his work. It is important to keep in mind that the most constructive suggestions in the world will be of no value unless they are acted upon. Two opposite reactions to criticism, neither of which is helpful, often occur. One way we may react is to become defensive and make excuses to justify our behavior; the other is to be completely submissive and outwardly accept whatever is said, even though the criticism seems to us to be unjust. In either case the final outcome is that all criticism or suggestions are rejected and we receive no benefit from the evaluation. People who react with excessive defensiveness or excessive submission are often people who are feeling threatened. When supervision is carried out in such a way that the worker does not feel threatened, extreme reactions will be diminished. We would hope to encourage a relationship in which the worker is able to admit his mistakes but at the same time feel free to speak in his own defense if he feels that a criticism is unjustified. Only on this basis can a truly cooperative, constructive supervisory situation exist.

A final word of caution about the nurse's responsibility in supervising co-workers is necessary. If the performance of the worker does not meet acceptable standards of nursing care after he has had an adequate orientation and a reasonable amount of teaching and supervision, it is the duty of the practitioner to report this fact to the proper person. Substandard practice or unsafe practice cannot be allowed to jeopardize the welfare of patients.

SELF-EVALUATION

The evaluation of learning is very closely bound up with the evaluation of teaching. If learning is not satisfactory, it may be due, of course, to some problem of the learner of which we are not aware or which we cannot remove; however, it may be due to unsatisfactory teaching. The nurse who sees the importance of teaching and wants to do a good job must take the initiative in appraising the teaching—that is, self-evaluation.

If it were possible to have an experienced teacher present at all our sessions of both formal and informal teaching and at evaluation conferences with our learners, we would have the great advantage of an objective point of view as well as an expert's opinion. Obviously, such an arrangement is not possible; therefore, it is the practitioner who must evaluate the teaching. Perhaps the most difficult problem in self-evaluation is maintaining objectivity.

We stressed earlier the problem of being subjective in the evaluation of our learners. Consider how much greater that problem becomes when we try to step to one side and watch our own performance. Generally, until we are able to attain at least some objectivity, we are likely to overrate or underrate ourselves; which way we rate ourselves is probably determined by the kind of people we are and how we see ourselves.

Clearly, neither overrating nor underrating ourselves is fair to us as teachers or to our learners. If we overrate ourselves and act accordingly, we will not examine ourselves and our teaching when learning is unsatisfactory, but instead blame the learners. If we underrate ourselves, we may become increasingly insecure and simply stop teaching, thus shrugging off an important responsibility of every nurse. Neither of these outcomes is justified—even the most experienced teachers make mistakes and the inexperienced teachers have assets they can build upon if these assets are recognized. The important thing is that the teaching which is part of our responsibility be done to the best of our ability.

In the process of evaluating our teaching, it can be helpful to get someone else's opinion if, in the first place, the person we ask has teaching ability and experience, and second, we pay attention to the comments we receive. Such a person should probably be someone we know professionally, rather than a personal friend. We are more likely to listen with at least some objectivity to a professional colleague and perhaps less likely to quickly rationalize out of existence the points that our colleague makes.

An important point to consider in self-evaluation is whether or not our learners are at ease with us. The importance of this question becomes clear when we recall that learning is affected by the emotional climate; that is, we learn better when we are comfortable in the learning situation. We could add a corollary here; we *teach* better when we are comfortable in the situation. If we really want to find out, it is not too hard to discover whether people are at ease with us: facial expression, body postures, changes in behavior when we approach—many signals tell us. It is not *necessary* for learning that student and teacher be at ease with each other, but it certainly helps.

Tape recording of class sessions can be a very revealing method of self-evaluation. During the process of teaching, particularly in group discussions, the nurse's attention is so taken up with what is going on that it is difficult to be completely aware of everything that is said at the moment or to recall it later. If a recording is made of the discussion, it can be played back after the class for purposes of careful study and self-evaluation.

If a tape recorder is available and the nurse is interested in using it for this purpose, there are several considerations to bear in mind. First, the learners should be told what the nurse's purpose is and asked if they are willing to have their voices recorded. There will generally be no objection and the initial self-consciousness of both the learners and the nurse will probably be quickly overcome. Second, the mechanics of recording must not interfere with the teaching. The group must be small enough to allow a stationary microphone to pick up the voices and tapes should not be rewound or changed during the class. Probably one side of a tape will provide enough of the discussion for evaluation. The play-back should be judged not only for evidence of the learners' response and the quality of their contributions, but also for the impression the nurse creates: the tone of voice, diction, choice of words, and the effectiveness of the questions asked and the explanation given. If this technique is used in an appropriate setting and the play-back is objectively evaluated, it can be an effective way of improving teaching.

The reader will find further material relevant to self-evaluation in Chapter 6 under discussion and demonstration as methods of teaching.

EVALUATING THE TOTAL TEACHING PROGRAM

Evaluation is essential for the success and continuing improvement of the total program. Evaluating the total program at regular intervals gives the practitioner a better perspective on what is being accomplished; day-to-day teaching has its successes and failures, sometimes attributable to the teacher, sometimes to the learners, sometimes to the teaching-learning situation or the difficulty of the material itself. Viewed in retrospect after several months, both the strengths and weaknesses of the program can be more objectively assessed and wiser decisions can be made if the need for change seems to be indicated.

Plans for program evaluation should be included as part of the general planning for teaching discussed in an earlier chapter. The nurse or nurses who are responsible for teaching are the key people to initiate and conduct the evaluation. The people who might be asked their views on the effectiveness of the program are the learners themselves, nursing supervisory staff, physicians, teachers in schools, supervisors in industry, and any other people who are interested in the program and are in a position to evaluate it. Nurses teaching in hospitals might get valuable suggestions from clinic or public health nurses who care for the patient after discharge.

Information might be obtained by the use of a simple questionnaire, by planned conferences, by noting comments made about the program in casual conversations. Where several practitioners work together in an agency, even though in different areas, much mutual benefit may be gained from sharing ideas and experiences and perhaps visiting each other's classes. Each nurse might assume responsibility for reviewing and updating a certain number of teaching guides at regular intervals, preferably at least once a year.

A word of warning is appropriate here, before we summarize: evaluation cannot be truly effective in improving teaching programs unless it is continual and consistent. It is relatively easy to make one all-out effort at evaluating the total program, particularly when everyone involved in the teaching program is doing the same thing; it is not so easy to take the initiative by oneself to continue painstaking evaluation from day to day. Although we said earlier in this section that evaluation at stated intervals has its advantages, it is the regular day-to-day evaluation by the practitioner that provides the information needed for the less frequent overall appraisals.

The specific methods and tools used to evaluate the teaching program as a whole will be determined by the particular circumstances existing in the nursing setting. As long as the end result is the continual strengthening and improving of the program, the fundamental objective of evaluation will be served.

SUMMARY

We have discussed various areas for evaluation and some of the pitfalls to be avoided. Evaluation is an integral part of the teaching process; it involves all aspects of learning and teaching. If it is viewed as a constructive process, it presents a challenge to the practitioner to evaluate effectively and consequently improve both teaching techniques and learning outcomes.

We have attempted throughout this book to emphasize basic principles and cite examples from the many settings in which nurses will carry out their teaching function—it remains for each individual practitioner to apply these principles, make modifications and adaptations to special situations, and continually evaluate the effectiveness of teaching and learning.

The successful accomplishment of the nursing practitioner's teaching function will bring satisfaction to the nurse and will contribute greatly to meeting the health needs of the members of our society.

REFERENCES

BOGUSLAWSKI, MARIE, et al. "Tape-Recording Patient Interviews: A Minimester Project." Nursing Outlook 17:41-45, May, 1969.
This article reports a project on patient interviews conducted by student nurses. The practitioner will note how much can be gained by taping any sort of session and studying the tapes at a later time.

GOLDSBOROUGH, JUDITH D. "On Becoming Nonjudgmental." American Journal of Nursing 70:2340-2344, November, 1970.
The author points out that everyone has judgmental feelings; what you feel is not as important as why you feel that way; when you know why, you can start to do something about it. The author shows some of the steps in becoming nonjudgmental.

GORDON, PHOEBE. "Evaluation—A Tool in Nursing Service." American Journal of Nursing 60:364-66, March, 1960.
This article, concerned with evaluation of all levels of nursing personnel by head nurses and supervisors, has relevance for the supervision of auxiliary workers by the practitioner.

REDMAN, BARBARA K. "Evaluation of Health Teaching," in The Process of Patient Teaching in Nursing. St. Louis: C. V. Mosby, 1968, pp. 106-26.
The author discusses the evaluation of the patient's learning and includes some aspects of written testing and various specific evaluation tools.

SCHWEER, JEAN E. Creative Teaching in Clinical Nursing. St. Louis: C. V. Mosby, 1968.
Although this book is directed to instructors in nursing programs, the reader will find the discussion of evaluation and evaluation techniques of value.

THOMAS, R. MURRAY. Judging Student Progress, 2d ed. New York: David McKay Company, 1960.
In the section of this book entitled "Understanding the Place of Evaluation," the author discusses the relationship of objectives and teaching methods to evaluation and presents a teacher's plan for evaluation.

YANKAUER, ALFRED, and others. "What Mothers Say About Childbearing and Parents Classes." Nursing Outlook 8:563-65, October, 1960.
This is a report of an interview survey of new mothers which includes their evaluations of classes for expectant parents and some suggestions for nurses who teach these classes.

Index

abstraction, 13
accepting the learner, 15, 28, 72, 118
acute illness, 43, 62-63
aggressive behavior, 30, 44, 45
assumptions *vs.* facts, 22, 32-33, 43
attitudes, teaching of, 11-12, 73

blackboards, 96-97
blind patients, communicating with, 9, 51-52
bulletin boards, 94-95

children in schools, 55, 56
    parents of, 56
chronic illness, *see* long-term illness
clients, defined, 2
communication, 31-32, 48-53, 81-82
    in supervision, 81-82
    language barriers in, 52-53
    non-verbal, 31-32, 51
    sensory deprivation and, 48-52
    verbal, 31-32
concept development, 12-15, 28, 87
    abstraction in, 13
    errors in, 13-14, 28
    generalization in, 13, 28
    integration in, 13
    perceptions in, 13
    through teaching materials, 87
    validation of, 14-15
    verbal symbols in, 12-13
conditioning, 9-10
    extinction of, 10
    process of, 9
    reinforcement of, 10
content, *see* subject matter
convalescence, 45-47, 63-64

courtesy, 30, 58
co-workers as learners, 2-3, 57-59
    age and experience of, 58
    defined, 2-3
    educational background of, 57-58
    in schools and industry, 58-59
    job security of, 58
    supervised by nurse, 57-58

deaf patients, communicating with, 9, 49-51
demonstration method, 11, 12, 77-80
discussion method, 74-77
displaying teaching materials, 94-97

emotions, 8-10, 12-17, 20-22
    effect of, on learning, 20-22
    effect of, on motivation, 15-17
    in concept formation, 12-15
    in conditioning, 9-10
    in perception, 8
employees in industry, 55
environment, control of, 37-38, 75
evaluation, 34, 39, 76-77, 80-82, 115-125
    and objectives, 34, 118
    attitudes toward, 81-82, 116
    by others, 122
    defined, 115
    frequency of, 124
    methods of, 118-121
    moral judgments in, 117-118
    of co-workers, 118-121
    of demonstration method, 80
    of discussion method, 76-77
    of specific lesson, 76-77, 80
    of total program, 123-125
    self-evaluation, *see* self-evaluation

127

expectant parents as learners, 55-56

failure in learning, 23
family members as learners, 54
filmstrips as teaching aids, 90
flannel or felt boards, 96
foreign-born learners, *see* non-English
   speaking learners

generalization, 13, 28, 43
group teaching, 47, 54-57, 74-80

habit formation, 22-23
halo effect, 117
handicapped learners, 52

imitation, 11-12, 73
independence, *see* self-help
informal teaching, 70-73, 84
integration, 13
interpersonal relationships, 27-30, 81-82
   in supervision, 81-82
interpreters, 52, 109-112

language barriers, 52-53
language cards, 53
laryngectomy patients, communicating
   with, 49-50
laws of learning, *see* principles of learning
learners in nursing settings, 24, 28-29,
   30, 36, 42-61
   as individuals, 28-29
   co-workers, 57-59
   need to give, 30, 44
   patients, 42-53
   people in good health, 54-57
   voluntary situation for many, 24, 36,
   42
learning, defined, 6
learning from the learner, 30, 44, 58
learning needs, 32-33, 103-104
   determining, 32-33
   predicting, 103-104
learning principles, *see* principles of
   learning
lesson plan, *see* teaching guide
listening, effective, 15, 20-22, 71-72
long-term illnesss, 43-45

magnetic boards, 96
methods of teaching, 11-12, 14-15, 20-
   22, 27, 70-86·
   asking and answering questions, 72-73
   demonstration, 11-12, 77-80
   discussion, 74-77
   informal, 70-73, 84
   setting an example, 12, 27, 73
   structured, 73-80
   supervision, 80-84

talking and listening, 14-15, 20-22,
   71-72
models as teaching aids, 89
moral judgments, 117-118
motion pictures as teaching aids, 90-91
motivation, 15-17, 23, 27, 45

non-English speaking learners, communicating with, 52-53, 109-112
non-verbal communication, 31-32, 51
nurse, nursing practitioner, defined, 1-2
nursing, 1, 2, 11, 12, 36, 42-43, 65-67,
   77-80
   functions, 1, 43
   priorities, 2, 36, 42-43
   procedures, performing, 11, 12, 66-67,
   77-80
   supportive care, 65-66

objectives, 33-35, 107, 111, 118
   clarification of, 33-35
   evaluation by means of, 118
   limitation of, 35
   purposes of, 33-34
   statement of, 35, 107, 111
objectivity in evaluation, 116-118
objects as teaching aids, 89
observation, 38-39, 83-84
   of other teachers, 38-39
   of the learner, 83-84
opportunities for teaching, 3-4
orientation to hospital, 8-9, 67-68
   new co-workers, 67-68
   patients, 8-9

pamphlets as teaching aids, 91-92
participation of learner, 18-19, 76, 79-80
patients as learners, 42-53
   in acute illness, 43
   in clinics or offices, 47
   in convalescence, 45-47
   in long-term illness, 43-45
   in the home, 47-48
patients with communication problems,
   48-53
   who cannot hear, 49-51
   who cannot see, 51-52
   who cannot speak, 49-50
   who do not speak English, 52-53
perception, 7-9, 12-13, 87
   defined, 7
   effect of disease on, 9
   errors in, 8
   in concept development, 12-13
   individual differences in, 8
   process of, 8
   teaching materials and, 87
pictures and photographs as teaching
   aids, 89-90

planning for teaching, 22-23, 33-37, 47, 74-80, 102-114
  completed teaching guide, 111-112
  developing program outline, 104-105
  in demonstration method, 77-80
  in discussion method, 74-77
  objectives in, 33-35
  overall program, 102-105
  outline for teaching guide, 106
  predicting learning needs, 103-104
  preparing teaching guide, 105-112
  time factor in, 22-23, 36-37, 47. 77
posters as teaching aids, 91-92
prejudices, 29-30
prevention of illness, 64-65
previous knowledge and experience of learners, 19-20, 57-58, 82-83
  determining, 19-20
  effect of, on learning, 19-20
  in supervision, 82-83
  of co-workers, 57-58
principles, 6-7
  application of, 7
  defined, 6
principles of learning, 7-25, 26, 38, 93
  application of, 7, 26, 38
  in programmed instruction, 93
  source of, 7
  summary of, 24
principles of teaching, 26-41
  source of, 26
  summary of, 39-40
programmed instruction, 92-93
promotion of health, 64-65

questions, 20, 32, 72-73

rapport see interpersonal relationships
readiness, 17-18
recordings, tape, 122-123
referrals, 23, 54
repetition, 22-23, 80
respect for the individual, 29-30, 45, 81

safety of patient, 19, 66-67, 80, 83, 84
satisfaction in learning, 23-24
school teachers as co-workers, 58-59
self-evaluation, 80, 120-123
  by learner, 120
  by practitioner, 80, 121-123
self-help, 3, 15, 30, 46-47, 63-64
sensory deprivation and its effect, 9, 48-52
  in communication, 48-52
  in perception, 9
setting an example, 12, 27, 73
slides as teaching aids, 90
sources of teaching materials, 97-100
  commercial, 100
  government agencies, 97-98

voluntary agencies, 98-100
stereotypes, 28-29, 43, 117
structured teaching, 73-80
students of nursing, 57
subjectivity in evaluation, 116-118
subject matter to be taught, 62-69
  in convalescence, 63-64
  in current illness, 62-63
  nursing procedures, 66-67
  orientation of new workers, 67-68
  prevention of illness, 64-65
  promotion of health, 64-65
  supportive nursing care, 65-66
supervision as teaching, 80-84, 118-121
  attitudes toward, 81-82
  cooperative relationship in, 81-82
  defined, 80
  evaluation in, 118-121
  knowledge of work and worker, 82-83
  observation in, 83-84
supervisors in industry as co-workers, 58-59
supportive nursing care, 65-66

talking, purposeful, 14-15, 20-22, 71-72
tape recordings, 122-123
teacher-made teaching aids, 92
teaching aids, see teaching materials
teaching, defined, 26
teaching function, 1-5, 42-43
  basic premise of, 4
  defined, 2
  factors affecting, 42-43
  importance of, 3
  opportunities for, 3-4
teaching guide, 105-112
  completed, 111-112
  outline of, 106
  preparation of, 105-112
teaching materials (aids), 87-101
  devices for display of, 94-97
  general considerations, 87-88
  sources of, 97-100
  types of, 89-94
teaching machines, 93
teaching methods, see methods of teaching
teaching principles, see principles of teaching
teaching skill, acquiring, 38-39
television as a teaching aid, 93-94
time, planning of, 22-23, 36-37, 47, 77
trial-and-error learning, 10-11, 80

verbal communication, 31-32
verbal symbols, 12-14
voluntary learners, 24, 36, 42

withdrawn behavior, 44-45